The people behind the book: Sam, Jo, Louise, Will, Harry, Vanessa carrying Felix and Oliver.

Introduction

This is a book that has taken four years to come about and about six months of hard slog to actually put together. When I first moved to Manchester, I found myself in a new city, with a new baby and a husband at work all day and I didn't know anyone. I promised myself this was a short term thing and we would be back down south within the year. Four years later I have come to love Manchester, made fantastic friends and it would have to take something pretty special to drag me back down the M6.

Babies in the City had been an idea in my head for so long (I even bought the domain name in 2004), but it was only when I became friends with Louise that it actually started taking shape and became a reality. She is the motivation behind the book and has kept things focused. Vanessa, a good friend and lawyer showed me some illustrations that she'd drawn for the book and suddenly it had an identity.

The initial idea was a guide for new mums; I was totally clueless about the best places to go with a newborn – where to breastfeed without feeling too self-conscious and where on earth were any baby changing facilities? As my children have got older and my needs have changed, so too has the book. It has evolved into a book also for mums with pre-school children, including classes and activities, hands-on museums and toddler friendly restaurants.

Every single entry has been road-tested and written by ourselves and other mums with Manchester mums in mind and with so many grandparents involved in the care of their grandchildren, this is essential reading for them too.

We have written the book based on our experiences. A lot depends on your child's mood and their likes and dislikes. Places do change and a great place can get worse and likewise, places can

get better. If your experience differs wildly from ours, please let us know. It is by no means an exhaustive list. There are still loads of attractions to visit which hopefully we will be able to include in next year's edition. There are probably places you love going and would recommend. Again we would love to hear about them.

Loads of friends have had an input and come up with quite a few of the ideas and locations in the book. They have also helped in putting it together, in particular Caroline and Shelley who have managed to read and check every word.

Lastly, we have to thank our partners, without them we could not have done nearly as much. They have picked up the slack, and even the odd child from nursery when we've forgotten. They've not only cooked dinner, but also bought it aswell. They have been dragged to various places around Manchester, (as have the children – but they didn't moan as much) and eaten in all types of restaurants. They have all been supportive and proud and offered advice and encouragement.

As we go to press Louise has less than four weeks to go until she has number two, so for any restaurants or museums who see a gorgeous blonde, perhaps a little tired, with a new baby and a notebook, beware – she'll be doing your review for next year.

For Louise, originally from Bolton and Vanessa from Bury, this book has been a nostalgic trip down memory lane visiting almost forgotten childhood favourites. For me, this is the book I wish had been available when I came to Manchester.

Jo Maxwell

Jo   Louise   Vanessa

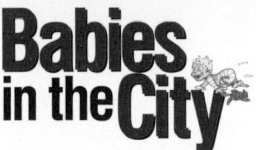

Babies in the City

Published by Babies in the City Limited
Unit 130, 792 Wilmslow Road, Didsbury, Manchester M20 6UG
Tel: +44 (0)161 438 2086
Email: info@babiesinthecity.co.uk
www.babiesinthecity.co.uk

Publisher: Jo Maxwell **Editor:** Louise Taylor
Cover Design & Illustrations: Vanessa Redmond
Production Editor: Shelley White
Sub-Editor: Caroline Blackburn
Contributors: Vanessa Redmond, Laura Halls, Fiona O'Sullivan,
Kathy Whitaker, Andrea Austin and Nuala Slim

This edition is first published in Great Britain in 2009 by
Babies in the City Ltd

ISBN: 978-0-9561215-0-9

A CIP Catalogue record for this book is available from the British Library

Printing and reprographics by Polestar Wheatons, Devon.

© Babies in the City Limited

Prices correct at the time of going to press. Where in operation, prices
include a voluntary 10% gift aid donation. Many places listed are
closed on Christmas Day and New Years Day. Opening times may be
different on bank holidays.

For each venue in Greater Manchester GMPTE have provided
information about the nearest bus, train or tram services and the stop
or station they use. We haven't identified specific services for places in
Central Manchester because you can easily get around the city centre
using Metrolink or free Metroshuttle buses (see Getting around
Manchester city centre on page 86).

DISCLAIMER
The publishers have made every effort to ensure the accuracy of
the information in this book at the time of going to press. However,
they cannot accept any responsibility for any loss, injury or
inconvenience resulting from the use of information therein. We
make no claims to pure objectivity in choosing our entries in this
book. The entries are here because we know of their existence
and/or have visited them or like them.

Our opinions and tastes are ours alone and this book is a
statement of them. We have done our upmost to get our facts right
but apologise if there are any mistakes. To the best of our
knowledge, all information is accurate as of the press date.

We do not check such things as fire alarms, kitchen hygiene,
health and safety regulations, CRB check compliance or any other
regulations which the owners of the entries in this book should
comply with as that is their responsibility.

OUT AND ABOUT

Museums and galleries

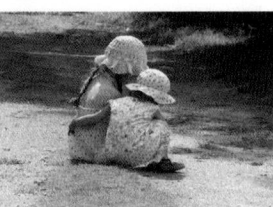

Parks, woods and walks

Contents

Museums and galleries

Manchester is brilliant for museums and galleries. Catering for all ages and tastes, there's arguably no better choice outside of London. Whether you're looking for a national centre of excellence like MOSI or a labour of love like the Museum of Transport, there's little doubt you'll be delighted with what you find.

Museums and galleries

Bolton Museum, Aquarium and Archive

This museum houses a diverse collection where you can get to know a little bit about the history of Bolton as well as visiting displays of art, egyptology, archaeology, botany and zoology. There's even an aquarium on the basement level with around 18 tanks of exotic fish to have a look at!

We spent the majority of our time in the museum section on the first floor. Exhibits included Samuel Crompton's Spinning Mule, a horse-drawn manual fire engine and antique toys. Climbing up the stairs to the balcony section we found a great collection of stuffed animals including a kangaroo, an enormous African elephant head, monkeys and eagles. Access with buggies or wheelchairs is possible using a private lift so contact a member of staff. Back downstairs we whiled away time in the large children's area. It's got books, a Noah's Ark, a puppet theatre and loads of nostalgic wooden toys and games.

Plenty of pre-school activities are held throughout the year so do check the website. Unfortunately there is no café or any kind of refreshments in the museum but there are shops and amenities very close by. Baby changing is on the ground and first floor. Ask at reception for access.

Mon-Sat 9am-5pm Admission free
Bolton Museum, Le Mans Crescent, Bolton BL1 1SE
Tel: 01204 332211 www.boltonmuseums.org.uk
Bus to: Bolton town centre. Train to: Bolton.

Central Art Gallery

This gallery is located upstairs in Tameside Central Library in a little gem of a building. We were lucky enough to go when both the gallery and library were hosting a Dr Who day, which was fabulous but unfortunately not a permanent exhibit.

With only two rooms displaying temporary exhibitions the gallery is small but friendly and welcoming. Noise and mess is encouraged and there is always a drawing table for all ages to create a piece of art. Regular children's activities for all ages are organised during the school holidays. Having experienced the Dr Who day, with its Dalek making table, I'm sure the activities would be fun and well structured.

Unfortunately there is no café, but there is a drinks machine in the library and some tables to sit at. We needed to buy some lunch during our trip so we went to nearby award-winning café and cake makers, Trifles, at 25-29 Market Avenue. It was a bit cramped with a pushchair, but we were allowed to park it by the doorway. The menu had appropriate choices for children and they offered smaller portions. The elaborately decorated cakes on display make good lunchtime viewing for children. So if you find yourself in Ashton-under-Lyne, perhaps visiting the market, and have an hour to spare, I would definitely suggest a visit.

Baby changing facilities are in the library.
Tues, Weds, Fri 10am-12.30pm/1-5pm,
Thurs 10am-12.30pm/1-7.30pm. Admission free
Sat 9am-12.30pm/1-4pm. Mon and Sun closed.
Central Art Gallery, Old Street, Ashton-under-Lyne
OL6 7SG Tel: 0161 342 2650
www.tameside.gov.uk/centralartgallery
Bus to: Ashton Bus Station. Train to: Ashton.

Eureka!

Voted by *The Independent* as one of the top three family days out in the UK in 2007, Eureka! is well worth the journey. Billed as the UK's National Children's Museum, the thousands of 'must touch' exhibits are designed to inspire children to find out about themselves and the world around them.

We ventured here during the half-term break and it was inevitably crowded (the website actually advises quieter times to be term time mid-week, sunny days and weekends in school holidays). It took us a long time to get in but once we were, it was fantastic and definitely worth the wait. Designed over two floors, there are six main galleries aimed at 0-11year olds and ranging from 'Me & My Body,' where you could find out what your skeleton looks like, to the 'Sound Garden', a giant sensory sound gallery for the really little ones with colourful singing flowers.

The favourite for our party was the 'Living & Working Together' section where the idea is that the children pretend they're grown-ups running the house and carrying out errands. You've got a scaled down Marks & Spencer store where the children shop with a little basket for their (fake) M&S food before scanning the products at a mini till; a Post Office where they could dress up in costumes and post various parcels and letters around the Town Square; a House with every room from the kitchen

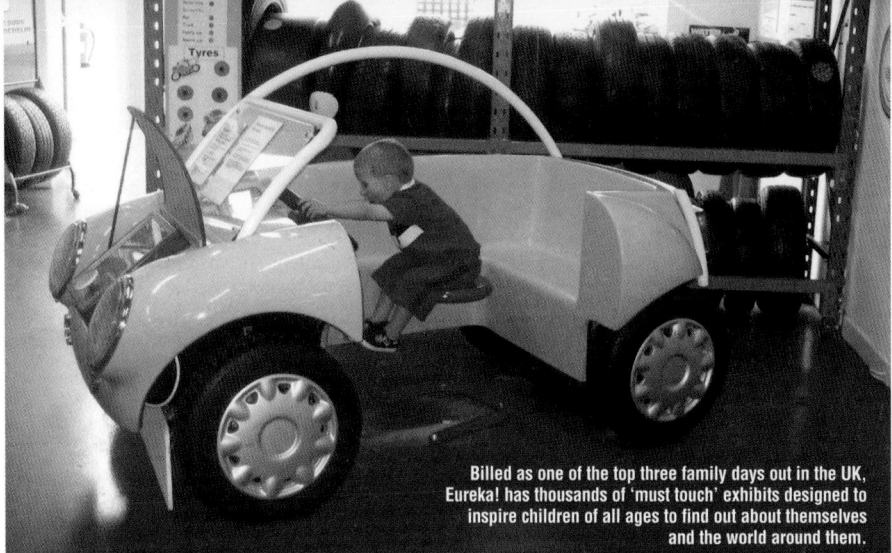

Billed as one of the top three family days out in the UK,
Eureka! has thousands of 'must touch' exhibits designed to
inspire children of all ages to find out about themselves
and the world around them.

to bathroom full of child-size props to explore; plus a fabulous Garage Workshop where there were miniature cars to sit in and steer, pumps to fill them with petrol, a car wash to manually operate and even a tyre changing bay.

The only snag came when we tried to get lunch. Lots of visitors meant the queues at the only café were enormous. Luckily one member of our group had had the presence of mind to pack a few snacks and drinks. So we took ourselves off to sit in the large heated railway carriage provided outside for those who bring their own lunch. That quickly filled up too, so, if you're struggling to find somewhere to plonk down, there are other seating spots on the second floor of the museum. Our advice is, if you are visiting at a busy time, take your own food.

Also worth noting are the pre-school activity room with arts and crafts for under fives and the large outdoor play area. Special events are held monthly at Eureka! in addition to the usual exhibition.
Mon-Sun 10am-5pm. Adult & Child from 3 years £7.25, Child 1-2 years £2.25, Under 1s free.
Buggy parks/toilets/baby changing on both floors.
Baby feeding room on first floor.
Eureka! The Museum for Children, Discovery Road, Halifax HX1 2NE
Tel: 01422 330069 www.eureka.org.uk
Bus to: Halifax town centre. Train to: Halifax.

Greater Manchester Fire Service Museum
The Fire Museum is a treasure trove of old fire engines, photographs and uniforms. Laid out as a Victorian street scene, it's really aimed at slightly older children, but there's still loads to look at and never underestimate the appeal of a big red fire engine to a small child. Whilst you aren't really allowed on the engines, once you get chatting to the

very friendly volunteers, they'll be happy to let you take a closer look (or at least they were with us).

Toilets and baby changing are available across the yard in the fire station. There is no cafe, but instead a coffee machine for 50p and crisps for 25p. Volunteers from the brigade have restored most of the exhibits and they also run the museum. It's only been open since January 2008 and already looks like it needs additional space. On the first Sunday of every month, the museum holds special events for families.

Parking wise, there is plenty on Richard Street, which is ideal as the entrance to the museum is here and not on Maclure Road. There is also a massive yard that they are happy for you to park in.
Every Fri and the first Sun of every month 10am-4pm. Admission free.
Greater Manchester Fire Service Museum, Maclure Road, Rochdale OL11 1DN Tel: 01706 901 227
www.manchesterfire.gov.uk/about-us/fire-museum.aspx
Bus to: Maclure Road/Tweedale Street (17, 471). Train to: Rochdale.

Greater Manchester Police Museum
Tucked away in the Northern Quarter of Manchester city centre is the Police Museum. Voluntary run, it's only open on Tuesdays. For toddlers I don't think it is worth a special trip, but if you're in the area and have an hour this is a lovely museum and it's free.

In the Transport Gallery there is a police car and bike for you to look at, but unfortunately not touch. There are a lot of glass cases containing police equipment and uniforms and a case filled with toy cars, which is what my children were most interested in. There are loads of dressing up clothes and handling items like police helmets, which are good fun. You can see the original charge office and the Victorian cells with wooden pillows, which gives

Museums and galleries

you a taste of prison life. Upstairs is a beautiful wood-panelled Magistrates Court dating from 1895.

There is a lift and toilets but no baby changing facilities. No refreshments are available, but you're not far away from city centre cafés. There is no car park but meter parking is available outside.

Tues 10.30am-3pm. Admission free.
GMP Museum and Archives, 57a Newton Street,
Manchester M1 1ET Tel: 0161 856 3287
www.gmp.police.uk/mainsite/pages/history.htm
Bus to: Manchester city centre. Tram to: Piccadilly Gardens.
Train to: Manchester city centre.

Hat Works – The Museum of Hatting

Hat Works is the UK's only museum dedicated solely to the hatting industry, hats and headwear. Set out over three floors, we headed to the first floor and this is probably the one best suited to under fives. The hundreds of hats are displayed in glass cabinets and though their attention wasn't held for that long, our three-year-olds really surprised us by taking quite a bit of interest. They liked the airline pilots' caps, old-fashioned firemen's helmets, frilly bonnets, rubber floral swimming caps and especially a native American head-dress. There's a large family fun area with hats to try on plus craft for the children to have a go at making their own – there are puzzles, puppets and a garage and cars to play with.

On the ground level, you'll find the machinery gallery. It's a recreated factory floor where you can see the collection of working Victorian style hatting machines along with a hatter's cottage and working

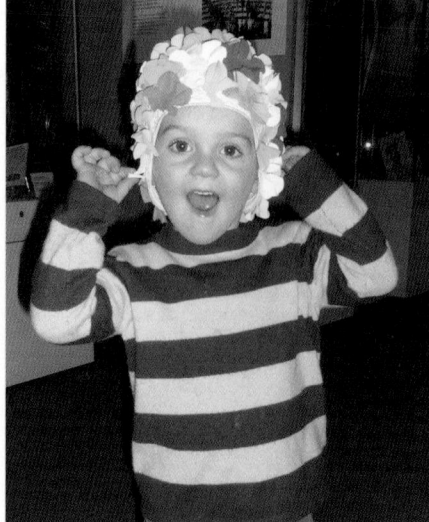

Hat Works – the UK's only museum dedicated solely to the hatting industry – has a large family fun area with hats to try on plus craft for the children to have a go at making their own.

office. Level 2 houses the café, shop and toilets with baby changing. There's lift access throughout.

Café Pure (run by a not-for-profit Stockport social enterprise) was excellent value for money. Hot snacks for adults include beans on toast for £1.95, with children's lunch boxes starting at £2.10 for four items.

There are two entrances to the museum – we used the A6 entrance (main reception and Level 2) and parked on Heaton Lane car park, which is just next to the viaduct – a 10 minute walk away. The second entrance brings you in on the ground level with the machinery gallery and is located on Daw Bank. Hat Works is also right next door to the bus terminal.

Mon-Fri 10am-5pm, weekends 1-5pm. Admission free.
Hat Works Museum of Hatting, Wellington Mill,
Wellington Road South, Stockport SK3 0EU
Tel: 0161 355 7770 www.hatworks.org.uk
Bus to: Stockport Bus Station. Train to: Stockport.

Imperial War Museum North

A morning trip to the Imperial War Museum lasted around an hour and a half, including a snack break. It is in a fabulous building and a great setting. The children loved the touchy feely action station and dressing up in the camouflage capes. The Time Stack interactive exhibits are probably more suited to older children, but staff are around to offer more information and take objects out for you to look at.

There are some brilliant large objects including a Harrier AV8 plane and a Russian tank outside (captured from Iraqi forces by the Royal Engineers in 2003), which of course the boys were desperate to climb on though unfortunately it's not allowed! I thought the Big Picture Show – the 360-degree film show projected on to the walls of the gallery – was excellent, but some children could be scared as the whole museum is thrown into darkness. They tend to run on the hour for about 15 minutes and they do give you a five-minute warning before it starts so that's the time to make a quick exit to the café.

There are also temporary exhibitions so check the website for the latest information.

The café is spacious with lovely views of the quay and a children's packed lunch costs £3.95. There are pens and paper available and the staff are happy to supply hot water to warm up milk or food. Toilets and baby changing facilities are downstairs, with the café and museum on the first floor (lift access throughout).

Car park £4. Admission free.
Mon-Sun 1st March-2nd Nov 10am-6pm,
Mon-Sun 3rd Nov-28th Feb 10am-5pm.
Imperial War Museum North, The Quays, Trafford
Wharf Road, Trafford Park, Manchester M17 1TZ
Tel: 0161 836 4000 www.iwm.org.uk
Bus to: The Quays (69). Tram to: Harbour City, then walk (across
the footbridge).

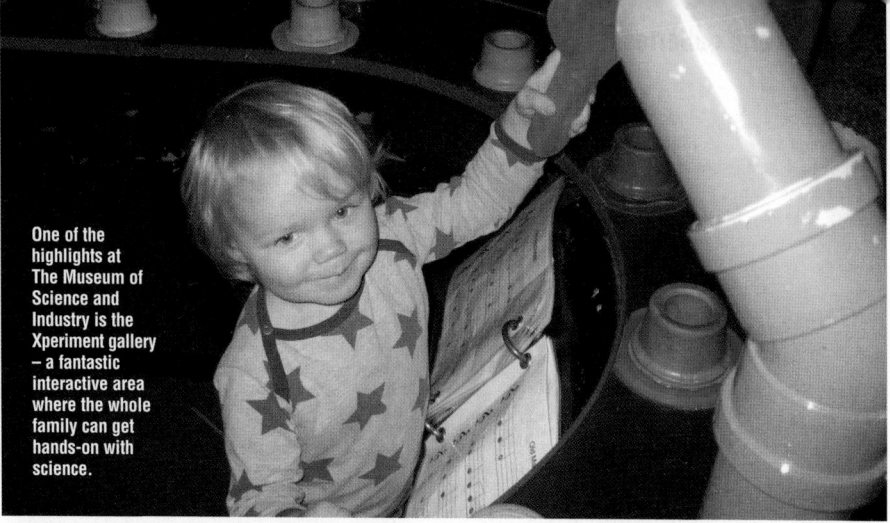

One of the highlights at The Museum of Science and Industry is the Xperiment gallery – a fantastic interactive area where the whole family can get hands-on with science.

MOSI – Museum of Science and Industry

MOSI is absolutely brilliant! It's pretty enormous, so my initial advice would be not to worry yourself trying to do everything in one trip – simply plan to come back again!

We started with the Air & Space Hall, which is in the building just across the road from the main entrance. It's full of planes, cars and motorbikes and the children loved having the freedom of space to run about. After this, it was on to the trains in the Power Hall, which also houses one of the largest collections of working steam mill engines in the world. Whilst we're on trains, worth mentioning is that outside you can take a ride behind a replica of Stephenson's Planet steam locomotive, which runs from April-October at weekends and during holidays 12-4pm (free for under fives). It can be cancelled at short notice so do check ahead before making a special trip.

Next up (or rather down) we went through the world's first passenger station in to the basement, where you'll find the Victorian Sewer (follow map if you need a lift). Built using original bricks from a Manchester sewer of the late 1830s, this is a real trip underground complete with smells and sounds. Admittedly our two-year-old was a little unsure but it's a great experience for those with less jittery children!

We ended up in the Xperiment gallery in the main building – a fantastic interactive area where the whole family can get hands-on with science. You can 'Lift the Mini' – using gears and chains, a real car travels up and down a vertical wall; pump the handle of the 'Water Wheel' to witness energy exchange; operate a 'Solar Mobile' – catching light using mirrors and tilting it onto solar panels suspended in the ceiling to make the mobile move. There are lots of tubes to shout down or smell; things to feel; writing with fibre optic lights; solving puzzles… quite simply, loads to have a go at! Another excellent element of Xperiment is the 'Discovery Den', a soft play area in one corner aimed at the under fives and filled with suitable toys.

When we eventually hit the Loft Café, the food selection was good and tasty. Children's portions of hot food started at £3.95 and on the day we were there Gorgonzola cheesy pasta and beef goulash were on the menu. A sandwich lunchbox costs £3.95 for five items. The café is big with plenty of highchairs and the staff will heat up baby food and bottles. There are also separate picnic areas if you choose to bring your own food. Baby changing is located throughout the main building and in the 1830 Warehouse. If you ask, staff will endeavour to find you a private room for breast feeding. Lockers are available on the ground floor.

Needless to say MOSI runs lots of special family events throughout the year so do check the website. A good one for the toddler set is Storytime – held every weekend and daily during holidays at 10.30am for 0-3 year olds lasting 20 minutes (it's free and you can just drop in). Also – Xperitots – activity sessions using puppets and storytelling for under fours, which takes place in the Xperiment gallery on the first Wednesday of every month, 10-11.30am. This costs £1 and must be booked in advance (note: whilst Xperitots takes place, the Xperiment gallery is closed to the general public). Finally, Engineer Eric's Difficult Day is a comical piece of theatre set in the Power Hall. Children get the chance to help Engineer Eric and Forgetful Fireman Fred start Pender, the Isle of Man locomotive. There's audience participation and lots of laughs. This free event is suitable for the over fours, starts at 12noon on weekends and holidays, lasts for 20 minutes and there is no need to book.

A visit to MOSI is a guaranteed success where kids are concerned. There's something for everyone and too much to cover in this entry – I didn't even get on to the Planetarium (minimum age advised six years) or the Textiles Gallery – you'll just have to go!

Car park £5 (£3 after 3pm). Meter parking close by.
Mon-Sun 10am-5pm
Admission free to permanent galleries.
Museum of Science and Industry, Liverpool Road, Castlefield, Manchester M3 4FP
Tel: 0161 832 2244 www.mosi.org.uk
Bus to: Manchester city centre and Metroshuttle 2. Tram to: G-Mex. Train to: Manchester city centre (nearest: Deansgate).

Babies in the City LOVE

Museums and galleries

The Lowry

Visiting The Lowry Galleries was a much more rewarding experience than I expected. First of all getting there – because it's slightly out of the centre and parking's all on site, it felt easy to access. There's also a bus service and the Metrolink tram drops you a 10-minute walk away. So we parked up and took a short stroll around the Salford Quays before arriving at the magnificent steel and glass clad Lowry building.

The feeling of space inside the brightly coloured foyer with its sloping blue floors is fantastic – we headed first for 'The Deck' and 'Family Corner', which are upstairs just to the left of the admissions desk. The Family Corner is aimed at the under fives and is a vibrant orange and red area full of mirrors, crayons and paper, magnet boards to stick things on and other games to play. The Deck area accommodates moving exhibitions. When we went, there was a display of amazing pop-up designs, where you could have a go at making your own and a comfy sofa with children's pop-up books to pore over.

Next, to the main gallery. Again it contains exhibitions that are continually changing throughout the year though there'll always be a collection of Lowry paintings on show. On our visit in the summer holidays, the exhibition was 'So you want to be an Artist?' and there happened to be lots of activities for children, which was great.

We ate at the Terrace Bar and sat outside overlooking the Ship Canal and Imperial War Museum – it was a perfect setting (there's also a restaurant serving similar food and a coffee shop with kids' lunch boxes). There are highchairs and a children's menu with four choices of meals such as fish bites and chips or pasta. It costs £5.95 for a main, dessert and a drink. The adult menu is quite extensive but not particularly cheap! A sandwich or salad starts at £5.75.

Baby changing facilities are available directly below the entrance foyer in both the ladies and gents toilets and there is a vending machine selling nappy and wipe kits for £1. Bottle and food warming facilities are by the Tower Coffee Shop. There are sloping floors and lift access to all levels.

Parking is in the Lowry Outlet Mall – it's free for four hours providing you make absolutely any purchase in the shops or restaurants – present your car park ticket at the till and staff will validate it.

Like many places, The Lowry offers lots of additional family activities aimed at pre-schoolers throughout the year, from dancing to messy art, so check the website.
Sun-Fri 11am-5pm, Sat 10am-5pm. Admission free. Food available 12-3pm and 5pm – 45minutes prior to curtain up.
The Lowry, Pier 8, Salford Quays, Manchester M50 3AZ

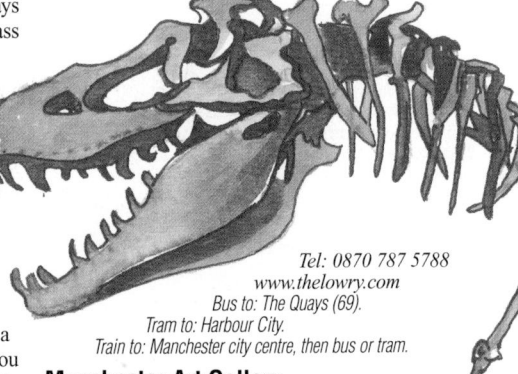

Tel: 0870 787 5788
www.thelowry.com
Bus to: The Quays (69).
Tram to: Harbour City.
Train to: Manchester city centre, then bus or tram.

Manchester Art Gallery

The Manchester Art Gallery was short-listed for the Guardian Family Friendly Museum Award in 2008. The gallery itself is of course stuffed with fabulous paintings by artists such as Adolphe Valette, Lowry and Turner, and while you're trying to check out the masterpieces there's a few dressing up clothes in various places for the children to play with.

We tried to encourage our two-year-old to follow the drawing trail (cartoon-esque labels underneath some of the paintings by the children's illustrator Tony Ross) around the gallery and despite him being a bit young for it, we had mild success! Another feature are the story play bags that you collect at the information desk (free, but deposit required). The ones for children aged 3-6 years contain things like novelty cushions, paper and pencils, a magnifying glass and farmyard animals. Even better there's the Clore Interactive Gallery on the first floor where you get to explore real works of art through a range of hands-on activities. There are computer screens with headphones where you press a button to choose the character you want to see and hear; a game where you can race chariots; and magnetic boards where you stick on various items like sink plungers to create your own portrait. It's definitely worth a visit.

We had a lovely lunch in the ground floor café. Food is served throughout the day (hot dishes 12-2.30pm). The children's menu had two hot dishes to choose from or a lunch box, all priced at £3.95. They were also given colouring packs. You can either buy baby food for 75p or bring your own and the staff will provide hot water to heat it up or a bottle warmer. Highchairs are available.

There are lifts to all floors or you can leave prams in the ground floor cloakroom. Baby changing is in both the men's and women's toilets on the ground floor next to the entrance hall. There are various car parks all within five minutes of the gallery.

The Mini Family Art Club for under fives runs the second Friday of every month 10.30-11.30am. Other free family events run throughout the year so contact the gallery for details of what's on.

Tues-Sun 10am-5pm. Closed Mon except Bank
Holidays. Admission free.
Manchester Art Gallery, Mosley
Street, Manchester M2 3JL
Tel: 0161 235 8888
www.manchestergalleries.org
Bus to: Manchester city
centre and
Metroshuttle 3.
Tram to: St. Peters
Square. Train to:
Manchester
city centre.

Manchester Museum

'Explore the world and travel through the ages' is what the blurb for Manchester Museum claims and it definitely delivers. It's impossible to describe this museum in just a few lines because its 15 galleries have a bit of everything. There's a skeleton of a sperm whale, an Egyptian room brimming with ancient art (including mummies) and Stan the Tyrannosaurus rex, among millions of other exhibits.

Highlights from our visit were the small but perfectly formed Vivarium and Aquarium where the snakes, lizards

and frogs entranced the children. We also got quite a lot out of the quaintly old-fashioned stuffed animal section, and the giant spider crab that welcomes you in the foyer is fantastic – it's over three foot high and nice and creepy!

A relatively new addition is the 'Play + Learn' space on the third floor where children can read, draw and relax. Close by is the picnic area if you have a packed lunch or alternatively there is the museum café, which is excellent. There's a well-planned children's menu with choices such as sausage and mash or fish pie for £3.50 (they're generous portions so sharing's an option) or you can get a lunch box for £4.50. Highchairs are available and staff will help with bottle and food warming for babies. Baby changing is throughout the museum.

Ultimately, it's a museum with a really nice feel and a wealth of exhibits. You can spend as little or as long as you like. Family orientated workshops are held regularly throughout the year so do check the website for details.

Tues-Sat 10am-5pm, Sun and Mon 11am-4pm.
Admission free.
The Manchester Museum, The University of
Manchester, Oxford Road, Manchester M13 9PL
Tel: 0161 275 2648 www.museum.manchester.ac.uk
Bus to: Oxford Road (15, 16, 41, 42, 42A, 43, 44, 46/47, 48, 111,
142, 143, 147, 191, 197, X57). Tram to: St Peters Square.
Train to: Manchester city centre (nearest: Oxford Road).

Museum of Transport

This is one that everyone should go to! The Museum of Transport is delightful. It's clearly a labour of love for all the volunteers that run it, and you can't help but be impressed by the enthusiasm behind it. Located within a genuine bus garage just off Cheetham Hill in Manchester, the museum features original transport offices preserved like time capsules from the past, complete with antique décor, furniture, old ticket machines and uniforms. Some of the collection was actually used in one of the Harry Potter films. There are over 70 restored buses, coaches and trams… honestly, when you first walk in, it's a sight to behold! You'll find yourself transported to a bygone age with vehicles dating from

Babies in the City LOVE

Museums and galleries

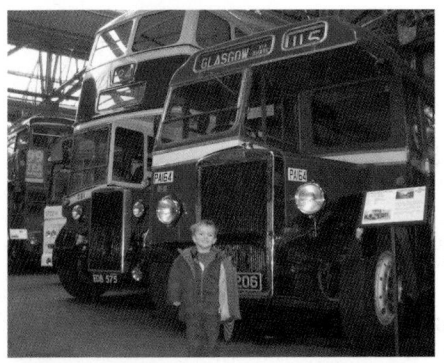

With over 70 restored buses, coaches and trams, when you first enter the Museum of Transport, it's a sight to behold. It really is a labour of love.

an elaborately painted Victorian open-top horse-drawn omnibus and a 1920s solid-tyred bus right up to the prototype for the modern trams that run in the city centre today, a few of which can even be climbed on.

Many of the buses are roadworthy and when the museum holds its frequent special event weekends (check the website), the classic buses are used to provide a free shuttle service, ferrying visitors to and from Victoria rail station or Heaton Park.

There is a café selling light refreshments including pies for £1.40 and a cup of tea for just 60p. They will provide hot water for heating up baby bottles. Baby changing is available in the disabled toilets and there is ramp access throughout the building.

Parking is on the road outside and we had no problems – one side has a yellow line so restrictions are in force weekdays and Saturdays until 12.30pm. The nearest car park is around five minutes' walk away at the Manchester Fort shopping centre.

Weds, Sat, Sun and Bank Holidays 10am-4.30pm.
The museum isn't free and depends on donations.
Adult £4, Under 16s £2, Under 5s free. Family ticket £10.
Museum of Transport, Boyle Street, Cheetham Hill,
Manchester M8 8UW
Tel: 0161 205 2122 www.gmts.co.uk
Bus to: Cheetham Hill Road (53, 59, 88/89, 135, 151, 167).
Tram to: Woodlands Road, then walk. Train to: Manchester city centre (nearest: Manchester Victoria), then bus.

Ordsall Hall

Ordsall Hall is a historic treasure – an amazing black and white half-timbered Tudor manor house located in the heart of Salford. It's a lovely place to visit with children as the exhibitions are very good, but it will be closing for two years around March 2009 for a massive restoration project.
Mon-Fri 10am-4pm, Sun 1-4pm.
Ordsall Hall, Ordsall Lane, Ordsall, Salford M5 3AN
Tel: 0161 872 0251 www.salford.gov.uk/ordsallhall
Bus to: Ordsall Lane (71, 73, 84, 92). Tram to: Exchange Quay.
Train to: Manchester city centre, then tram.

Salford Museum and Art Gallery

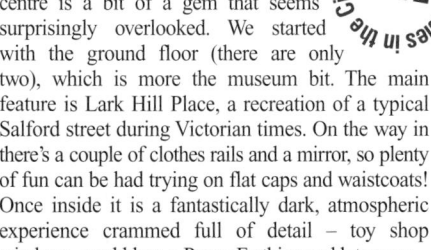

This small museum and gallery on the A6 approach to Manchester city centre is a bit of a gem that seems surprisingly overlooked. We started with the ground floor (there are only two), which is more the museum bit. The main feature is Lark Hill Place, a recreation of a typical Salford street during Victorian times. On the way in there's a couple of clothes rails and a mirror, so plenty of fun can be had trying on flat caps and waistcoats! Once inside it is a fantastically dark, atmospheric experience crammed full of detail – toy shop windows, a cobblers, a Penny Farthing and lots more.

The art galleries are upstairs and the Victorian Gallery in particular contains plenty of activities to keep all ages amused whilst you take in some art. There is colouring, sculptures to touch, worksheets full of quizzes such as matching up the animals on the sheet with the animals in the paintings, and a box with hats in that again link in with the pictures. Most successful for us however were the colourful soft bags placed strategically round the room that contained various items relating to the paintings they were under. For example, the portrayal of Queen Victoria's arrival in Salford has a bag underneath containing crowns, books, a flag and a mini ermine and fur robe. It is a really well thought out idea.

The LifeTimes Gallery hosts changing exhibitions focusing on different aspects of Salford's history over the last 200 years. One recent theme was music, when a corner of the room was dedicated to children with a miniature record shop (complete with till and vinyl singles) and small musical instruments to play on. A definite hit with the under fives.

We had a quick cup of tea in the Lark Hill Tea Shop (open Mon-Fri 10am-3.30pm, Weekends 1-4pm) and although there's not a dedicated children's menu, we thought the food on offer sounded good value – sandwiches and toasties from £2.00. Highchairs are available and staff will heat up baby bottles and food. Baby changing's in the disabled toilet on the ground floor – you need to get the key from reception which is close by.

Salford offers additional family-friendly exhibitions throughout the school holidays. It also advertises 'Gallery Tots', a once-a-month story, singing, games and craft session for pre-schoolers.

Free parking is in front of the museum. Salford Crescent train station is a five-minute walk away.
Mon-Fri 10am-4.45pm, weekends 1-5pm. Admission free.
Salford Museum and Art Gallery, Peel Park,
The Crescent, Salford M5 4WU
Tel: 0161 778 0800 www.salford.gov.uk/museums
Bus to: Salford Crescent (8, 12, 26, 31, 32, 36, 37, 67, 68, 100, X34, X61). Train to: Salford Crescent.

Staircase House

This is a modern museum set in the oldest house in Stockport. It is a rare place indeed that actively encourages children to climb on the beds, touch everything and dress up in the various clothes dotted around, but that is exactly what's on offer.

On arrival children are handed a cloth activity pack with individual mini-bags numbered to the relevant rooms. Do not get one for each child, it takes three people to manage this; one to hold the big bag, one to get the stuff out and the other to control the children! Inside there is also a laminated sheet which basically tells you the same thing; the packs are aimed at older ones but it is worth getting one just for the two glove puppets that are included.

In all the rooms bar the dining room children are encouraged to inspect, touch and play with the objects, which gives you time to have a good look round yourself. One of the favourites for the under fives is the counting room, where you can write with quill pens and literally get covered in ink. Another is the dressing up area – the only downside is that it is hard to drag them away.

Being linked to a modern building means that Staircase House has all the essentials, including a lift and baby changing facilities. The Stockport Story Museum is also housed in the modern section and gives a background to life in the town. It is a little bit dry for children but is definitely worth a look. There is a toy box at the bottom level that does gain you an extra 10 minutes while they take a root through.

Parking is fine on a Sunday as there are single yellow lines outside the building. During the rest of the week there is a pay and display car park nearby.

Staircase House: Mon-Fri 12noon-5pm, weekends and Bank Holidays 10am-5pm.
Adult £3.95, Under 5s free.
The Stockport Story Museum: Mon-Sun 10am-5pm.
Admission free.
Staircase House, 30-31 Market Place, Stockport SK1 1ES.
Tel: 0161 480 1460 www.staircasehouse.org.uk
Bus to: Stockport town centre. Train to: Stockport.

TOP FIVE MUSEUMS AND GALLERIES

MOSI
Literally a powerhouse! The best museum of its kind in the UK – there's something for everyone.

Museum of Transport
Remember the days when a bus was a thing of beauty, well here are over 70 restored buses, coaches and trams – honestly, when you first walk in, it's a sight to behold.

Manchester Art Gallery
Loads to see and do for the whole family, from dressing up games to chariot racing, at this award-winning city centre art gallery.

Eureka!
The UK's National Children's Museum. Voted one of the top three family days out in the country, Eureka! is well worth the journey.

Salford Museum & Art Gallery
A bit of a gem that's definitely worth discovering. Stroll down its recreated Victorian street with authentic period shops – a must for adults and children alike!

Stockport Air Raid Shelters

Stockport Air Raid Shelters is a network of tunnels nearly a mile long, dug out of the soft red sandstone hills on which Stockport town centre stands. We went on a Friday just after the last school trip of the day, so we had the tunnels to ourselves. We were specifically asked at reception if our three-year-old would be ok with the audio-visual display. They warned us it was quite loud. I thought he would be fine but he wasn't! The lights went down, the sirens started and Will freaked – we were back in the reception area within 30 seconds!

The labyrinth of tunnels are remarkable, authentically restored with props that give you a taste of daily life in 1940s war-torn Britain. The tour is very well illuminated and fully accessible for wheelchair users. The Air Raid Shelters are perhaps more suited to older children but it really does depend on the type of child you've got! There is no café or refreshments, no toilets or baby changing facilities, although there are public toilets directly across the road. There is some metered parking outside or Merseyway multi-storey car park a minute away.

Mon-Sun 1-5pm (last admission 4pm).
Adult £3.95, Under 16s £2.95, Under 5s free.
Stockport Air Raid Shelters, 61 Chestergate, Stockport SK1 1NE
Tel: 0161 474 1940 www.airraidshelters.org.uk
Bus to: Stockport bus station. Train to: Stockport.

Staircase House is rare in that it positively encourages children to climb on the beds and touch everything!

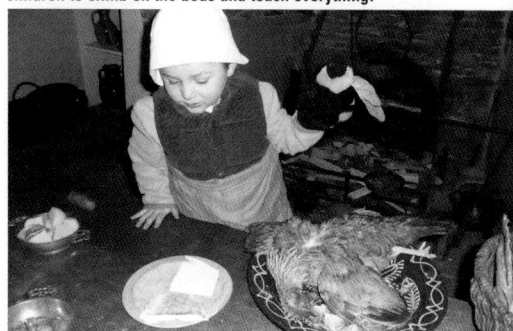

Museums and galleries

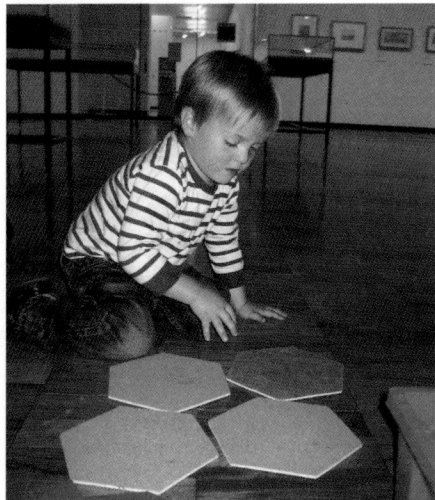

A visit to the Whitworth Art Gallery is a perfect antidote to a rainy day.

Tate Liverpool

The gallery itself, whilst terrific for adults, isn't geared for children. But if you can get an hour while your child is asleep in the pushchair, it's a lovely place to visit. The art is world class and the building is very pram friendly with ramps and lift access throughout.

The café has a selection of good and wholesome choice for the adults – exotic sandwiches, salads, pastas and dips. The children's menu has a choice of fish fingers, pasta or a cheese sandwich with cucumber and carrot sticks. This is topped off with fruit salad, chocolate brownie or banana split and washed down with fruit juice. It's a pretty good deal at £4 and that includes crayons and a colouring sheet. There are plenty of highchairs and a unisex baby changing facility in the basement below the café.

If you are visiting with toddlers this is an ideal trip to combine with The Yellow Duckmarine, otherwise known as the Wacker Quacker. This is a fleet of World War Two amphibious vehicles painted bright yellow and used to provide guided tours around the city. The tour guides are jokey and informal and the vehicle is unusual enough, what with its roll-up polythene windows etc to keep young minds and hands occupied. However, all of this pales into insignificance compared with the moment when children realise the bus is actually going to drive into the river. You hurtle down the gangplank arriving with a huge splash, the tour finishs with a half-hour motor round the docks.

Tours depart approximately every hour, seven days a week from 10.30am till dusk (lasting around an hour). The ticket office opens at 9am. Children under two must sit on an adult's lap and only two babies are permitted on each tour. Prams and pushchairs can be left in the ticket office by the Albert Dock Visitor Information point.

The Yellow Duckmarine, 32 Anchor Courtyard, Albert Dock, Liverpool L3 4AS
Tel: 0151 708 7799 www.theyellowduckmarine.co.uk
Adult £9.95, Child £7.95, Under 2s free.
School Bank Holidays, weekends Mar-Sept
Adult £11.95, Child £9.95, Under 2s free.
Tate Liverpool, Albert Dock, Liverpool L3 4BB
Tel: 0151 702 7400 www.tate.org.uk/liverpool
Tues-Sun Oct-May 10am-5.50pm (closed Mondays).
Mon-Sun June-Sept 10am-5.50pm.
Admission free apart from special exhibitions.
Train to: Liverpool Lime Street. Bus to: S1 The City Centre Circular Route to Albert Dock.

The Whitworth Art Gallery

A visit to the Whitworth is a perfect antidote to a rainy day. If you're still with a pushchair it's very easy to get around, plenty of ramps – and just over two floors. Admittedly if you're with a toddler you're not going to be able to spend all day there but we happily passed away a couple of hours. Not only that, it's ideal if you simply fancy a delicious lunch with some friends.

There's a fantastic children's corner on the ground level. It's furnished with bean bags and cushions for the children to sprawl about on and an 'art cart' filled with a multitude of activities such as jigsaws, sticklebricks and giant floor shapes. Dotted around the gallery are activity stations with hats to try on, outfits to climb into and colouring pencils. Every Sunday from 1.30-3.30pm the Whitworth runs 'Colourful Sundays' – a free drop-in suitable for all ages where you can have a go at making things such as robot head masks! All year, but particularly during the school holidays, the Whitworth is very proactive in putting on specific family events and art workshops for all age ranges, so it's worth checking the website or calling in for a leaflet about what's coming up.

We ate at the award-winning Gallery Café and were suitably impressed. The menu's nice and seasonal, the food's clearly freshly-made and there's always a children's option available – the day we went it was houmous and carrot sticks with a chicken sandwich, which was £5 including a drink and a brownie. Staff at the café are also more than happy to provide hot water to heat up jars and bottles. Baby changing facilities are available in the unisex disabled toilet on the ground floor. If you want to take a packed lunch there are picnic tables outside and a large grassy area as well as Whitworth Park next door.

12 **Babies in the City**

Museums and galleries

My final tip is that as the gallery's positioned on a busy bus route, you may want to think about combining a visit with a bus trip for your toddler. If you're driving, it is worth trying to grab a free place on Denmark Road next to the gallery, although there is a two-hour time limit imposed. Otherwise there's a couple of car parks signposted just across the road.

Mon-Sat 10am–5pm, Sun 12noon-4pm. (Note: due to a major exhibition installation in 2009, there may be days the gallery is closed so it is advisable to check before going). Admission free.
The Whitworth Art Gallery, The University of Manchester, Oxford Road, Manchester M15 6ER
Tel: 0161 275 7450 www.manchester.ac.uk/whitworth
The Gallery Café at The Whitworth serves breakfast Mon-Sat 10-11.30am, lunch 12noon-4pm,
Sun 12noon-3.30pm. Open for drinks until later.
Bus to: Oxford Road (15, 16, 41, 42, 42A, 43, 44, 46/47, 48, 111, 142, 143, 147, 191, 197, X57). Tram to: Piccadilly Gardens, then bus. Train to: Manchester Oxford Road, then bus.

Touchstones Rochdale

Based alongside the Tourist Information Centre in Rochdale, Touchstones is a modern, well laid out arts and heritage centre. It is ideal for under fives as there is just enough to keep their interest and I stayed much longer than I'd planned.

Although the museum is all in one room, the space is really well utilised as you keep noticing new things. There are loads of interesting objects accompanied by manageable amounts of text.

My three year old, after much persuading, enjoyed crawling through the coal pit tunnel and there were lots of hands on activities in drawers including a bucket which smelt disgusting when you took the lid off, plus a lovely area with dressing up clothes and a large mirror.

There is a small but enticing café attached to the museum that offers good value options such as a bacon bap and cup of tea for £2. They also have heaps of cakes and do children's lunchboxes for £3.50. Baby changing is in both the ladies' and disabled toilets on the ground floor and there is lift access to the art gallery.

I left Touchstones with a real sense of times gone by in Rochdale; the staff were helpful and friendly and all told it was a thoroughly enjoyable visit. There is pay and display parking immediately outside and I'm glad I'd put in £1 for two hours instead of 70p for an hour.

Mon-Sat 10am-5pm, Sun and Bank Holidays 12noon-4.30pm. Admission free.
Café: Mon-Sat 11am-4pm.
Touchstones Rochdale, The Esplanade, Rochdale OL16 1AQ
Tel: 01706 924492 www.rochdale.gov.uk
Bus to: Rochdale town centre. Train to: Rochdale.

Urbis

Since its arrival in 2002, Urbis has gone on to form an iconic part of Manchester's skyline. It's essentially an exhibition centre about city life showcasing contemporary art and design and Manchester's popular culture. We took advantage while our little one was asleep to enjoy one of the exhibitions. When he woke up a few rides in the wonderful glass elevator appeased him greatly.

For those with older children Urbis Learning runs a wide range of family activities throughout the year.

We've also popped our heads in on the odd Saturday when inevitably traipsing round shops has proved too much for our toddler. Urbis run an arts and craft table for children of all ages every weekend. Often influenced by the current exhibitions, it runs from 12-3pm, costs £1-£3 per child and there is no need to book.

The Social is the newly refurbished café within Urbis. See page 63 for more information.
Jan-June, Tues-Sun 10am-6pm; June-Sept, Tues and Weds 10am-6pm, Thurs-Sat 10am-8pm, Sun 10am-6pm; Sept-Dec, Tues-Sun 10am-6pm Admission free
Urbis, Cathedral Gardens, Manchester M4 3BG
Tel: 0161 605 8200 www.urbis.org.uk
Bus to: Manchester city centre and Metroshuttle 2.
Tram to: Victoria.
Train to: Manchester city centre (nearest: Victoria).

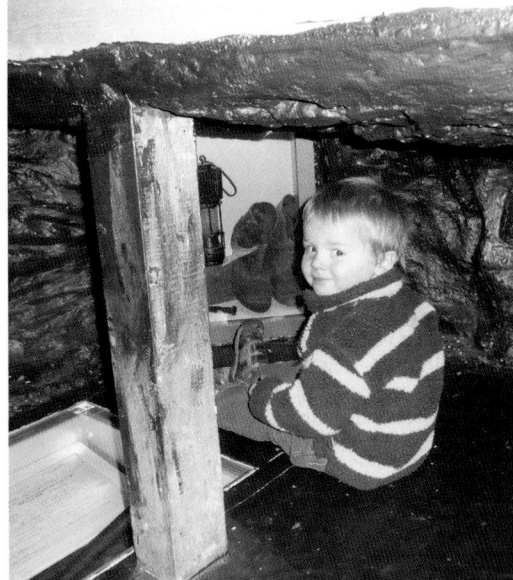

Touchstones is a modern, well laid out arts and heritage centre that is ideal for the under fives. Sam took some persuading to crawl through the model coal mine.

Parks, woods and walks

Don't be deceived by the relative lack of city centre parks in Manchester. You're within easy reach of the grandeur of the Peaks and Pennines; the wildlife and woodlands along the Mersey Valley and the faded Victorian glamour of Heaton and Vernon Parks. So unpack your wellies and take to the great outdoors.

Parks, woods and walks

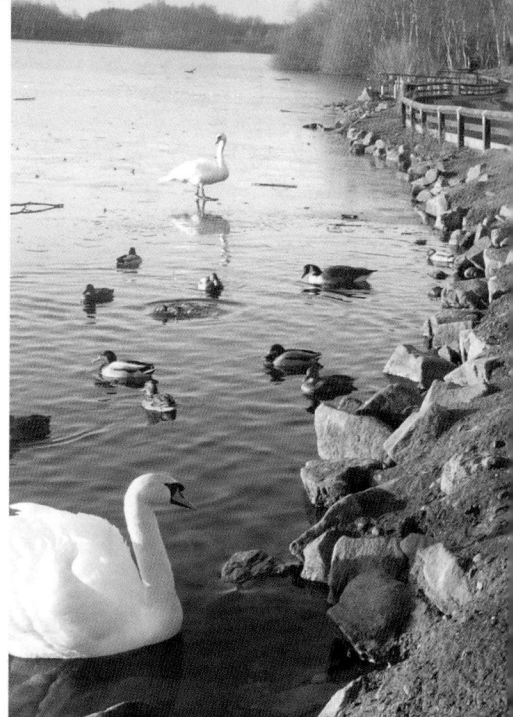

Alderley Edge

Alderley Edge is a National Trust woodland with an impressive sandstone escarpment (the Edge!) and spectacular views over Cheshire country-side to the Peak District. It's a place steeped in mystical folklore – King Arthur and his men are said to sleep beneath the cliffs, and the area is strongly associated with a wizard thought to be Merlin.

We always have fun at Alderley Edge: with plenty of woodland tracks to explore and tree trunks to climb it's not surprising. We usually follow the wizard's walk, a 3.5 mile route taking in a number of landmarks featured in the legend of the wizard. Not for the faint hearted is the 'thieves hole' – a very deep unlit circular cave dug into the red sandstone high enough to walk into. My four year old thinks it is marvellous and dares himself to go deeper and deeper into the darkness before fright gets the better of him. Elsewhere you'll find a water pump to mess with; a tiny wizards house (a stone hut!) and the Beacon marking the highest point of the Edge. Whilst this is great to climb up to, some of the paths are a bit steep. We've managed with a pushchair but you can avoid them if you wish.

The Edge itself (which can be accessed from the wizard's walk) is amazing for the views and there are nooks and crannies to climb in, but do be careful as there are a few high and sheer drops around this area. Hopefully you might stumble across one of the popular tree trunks that you can climb. They're in a clearing in the woodland; one forms an arch from the ground to about adult head height; people take turns to try and cross it. My two children make it a third of the way across – holding a hand. Daddy has helped down one or two petrified children who have gone too far, to say nothing of myself for that matter!

If you are stuck for something to do on those perpetual rainy days but feel like getting some fresh air, then try Alderley Edge. The woodland canopy is dense enough to provide shelter from the rain during the spring and summer months.

There's also a tea room and a small enclosed wooded picnic area with tables, or alternatively you're not too far from a pub for stronger refreshments. More importantly to my children is the ice-cream van regularly situated in the car park. It always encourages them to 'walk' those last few metres back! There is an information office selling maps of walks (although some of the walks are signed), and children's quiz/trails. Public toilets are in the car park but provide no baby changing.

Access to the Edge: Winter 8am-5.30pm,
Summer 8am-6pm
Tea-room: Weekends Winter 10am-5pm,
Summer 10am-6pm and Bank Holidays
Admission free. The car park is pay and display, but is free to NT members.
Alderley Edge, Situated on B5087 at Nether Alderley, Macclesfield, Cheshire SK10 4UB Tel: 01625 584412
www.nationaltrust.org.uk

Boggart Hole Clough

Boggart Hole Clough is an ancient, densely wooded park three miles north of Manchester city centre. Park in the free Charlestown Road car park and set off in the direction of the lake. The park is anything but flat...! As the name indicates it's in a clough – which means a ravine. In former times, the clough was said to be haunted by the Boggart, a mischievous goblin or phantom.

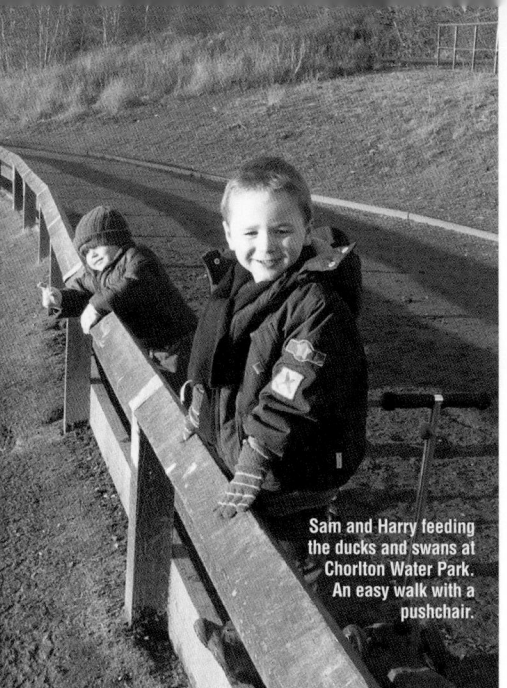

Sam and Harry feeding the ducks and swans at Chorlton Water Park. An easy walk with a pushchair.

Bruntwood Park

The best reason for visiting Bruntwood is its modern and well-equipped playground. There are three areas side by side, each aimed at different age groups. All the usual swings, slides and roundabouts etc are present, plus a really big climbing frame with lots of interesting bits and one of our favourites, the giant ball catcher – where you hurl your ball into a large metal bucket on a 7ft high pole and wait for it to drop out of one of four holes.

The different play areas are linked by gentle slopes which are perfect for children learning to ride a bike. In season and during most school holidays there's an inflatable bouncy castle (you do have to pay though). There's also vast expanses of green grass, mature woodland, ponds (with ducks) and wetland areas to explore.

Attached to Bruntwood Hall (not open to the public), in the original Victorian conservatory there's The Vinery restaurant. It's very child friendly (lots of highchairs and they will heat bottles and jars). For children you can choose things like pasta, sausages, fish fingers or sandwiches and together with a drink and ice cream you'd be paying £3.20-£3.50.They also serve breakfast which is handy for early risers! Baby changing facilities are in both mens and ladies toilets.

Back in the park, there's outside seating and a refreshment kiosk open weekends and holidays. There is a baby changing room in the toilet block close to the kiosk.

The Vinery: Winter 10am-4pm,
Easter onwards 10am-5pm Tel: 0161 491 0531
Bruntwood Park, Bruntwood Lane, Cheadle, Stockport SK8 1HX
Tel: 0161 428 5391 www.stockport.gov.uk
Bus to: Schools Hill (312), Cheadle Road (130, X57, 309/310)
Train to: Cheadle Hulme, then bus.

We were a bunch of one pram containing baby, one toddler walking and three on scooters. So the scooters were whizzing perilously down hills, the mum with the pram was puffing up hills and amazingly the toddler just kept on walking regardless! We found the lake and had a walk round – it's nice enough but a bit neglected. You could imagine how it was in its glory days. We then headed further downhill into a more wooded section which made for a picturesque walk (there are tarmac pathways throughout so prams aren't a problem if you can cope with the ups and downs). We were aiming for the playground at the Rochdale Road end of the park, which was probably about a half hour child's walk from the lake. This playground when we got there turned out to be a bit bleak. You'd be better going to the other one close to Charlestown Road car park which is relatively new and has swings, climbing activity train and a cup roundabout.

Toilets are at the main car park. They're accessed by key kept in the adjacent visitor centre (Mon-Fri 8am-4.30pm, weekends warden dependent). No baby changing. There are plans to install a café in the old boathouse on the lake in 2009.

Boggart Hole Clough, Charlestown Road, Blackley, Manchester M9 7DF
Tel: 0161 795 2650 www.manchester.gov.uk/leisure
Bus to: Charlestown Road (51, 118) Rochdale Road (16, 17, 64, 123, 124, 131, 163). Train to: Manchester city centre, then bus.

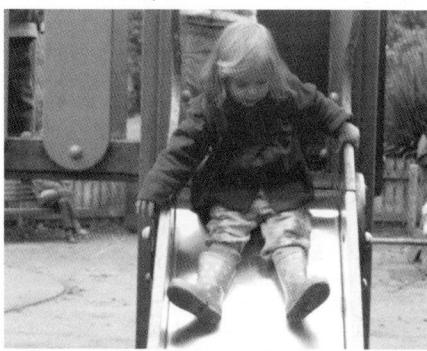

The best reason for visiting Bruntwood Park is its modern and well-equipped playground. There are three areas next to one another aimed at different age-groups.

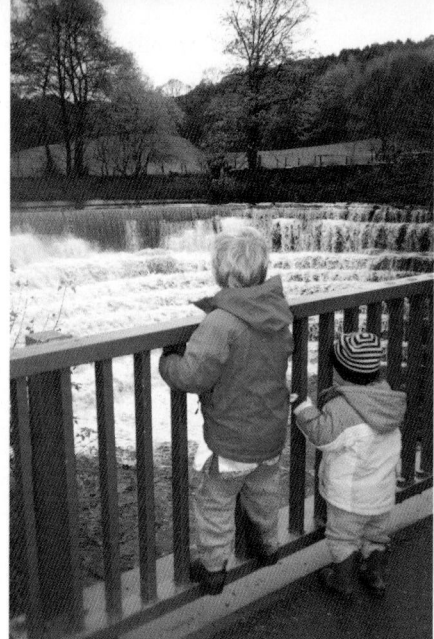

At Etherow Country Park the circular walk to the weir and then round the lake took just over one hour fifteen minutes. For a picnic there are tables overlooking the weir.

Chorlton Water Park

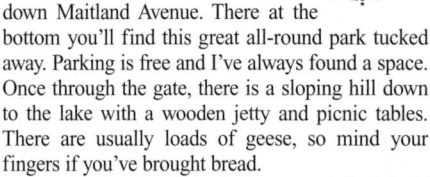

When I first arranged to meet friends at Chorlton Water Park I almost missed the little blue sign directing you from the main road down Maitland Avenue. There at the bottom you'll find this great all-round park tucked away. Parking is free and I've always found a space. Once through the gate, there is a sloping hill down to the lake with a wooden jetty and picnic tables. There are usually loads of geese, so mind your fingers if you've brought bread.

I tend to head anti-clockwise around the lake if I'm trying to get the little ones to walk or scooter avoiding the playground until the end. It is a very easy one mile walk with paved paths, great for pushchairs or bikes. There are a couple of gentle sandy slopes down to the lake, ideal for feeding the ducks or poking around in the mud with a stick.

If you're prepared to explore, take little detours off the path and you'll find great blackberry bushes and almost directly across the lake from the main entrance, over the bridge you'll discover a path on your left leading to Kenworthy Woods – essentially a secret orchard, offering apples, plums and pears and you're welcome to help yourself.

There's not a lot in the playground – in truth it's probably due a revamp. To the right, through the trees is an Education pond with a boardwalk, so be careful with toddlers.

There is no café but if you've got an off-road buggy and fancy a more strenuous walk, the River Mersey runs alongside the park, so you can join the Transpennine trail and head to Sale Water Park for a coffee, approx 2kms. On fine days there is also an ice cream van that does a great trade.

Toilets are in the car park and the disabled toilet does have baby changing facilities but you'll need to get the key from the office. The office is open during normal working hours and at the weekend there is an information desk open 9.30am-12noon.
Chorlton Water Park, Maitland Avenue, Chorlton, Manchester M21 7WH
Tel: 0161 881 5639 www.merseyvalley.org.uk
Bus to: Barlow Moor Road (23, 23A, 46, 47, 86, 270). Train to: East Didsbury or Manchester City centre, then bus.

Clifton Country Park

Clifton Country Park boasts over 50 hectares of perfect meadows, woods, ponds and lakes and is a very appealing tranquil setting. The main car park is by the visitor centre with a children's playground on your left hand side just before you reach the water's edge. The play area's suitable for 3-11 year olds with the usual swings, slides, rope bridge and climbing frame. There's an equestrian centre close by, so horses are in the fields for toddlers to have a look at.

The main lake is huge, with geese and swans eagerly waiting to be fed and a purpose built jetty to get to them. It's surrounded by buggy friendly stone surfaced paths and took me about 40 minutes to walk round. It's mostly flat with lots of benches for resting and is well maintained. There's no café, but often a van sells refreshments in summer. Baby changing is available in the toilets situated in the visitors centre but this isn't all the time. 'Buggy walks' and various children's activities are held regularly, so do get in touch with the visitors centre for more details. What appealed to me was the Tree Trail – some very user-friendly leaflets (pick up at the centre) with clear photographs of assorted leaves and the name of their respective trees for the older children to spot along the way.
Visitor centre: Sun 10am-5pm, Mon-Tues 1-5pm (these hours can be slightly unreliable during the winter).
Clifton Country Park, Clifton House Road, Clifton, Salford M27 6NG Tel: 0161 793 4219
www.salford.gov.uk/cliftoncountrypark
Bus to: Manchester Road (8, 22). Train to: Manchester, then bus.

Daisy Nook Country Park

Daisy Nook is an area of the Medlock Valley between Oldham, Failsworth and Ashton under Lyne. Despite us missing the turning it is actually quite easy to find (follow the sign to Daisy

Nook Garden Centre) and is only five minutes from the motorway and Ikea. At the bottom of the hill is a free car park and The John Howarth Countryside Centre, a visitor centre with displays and murals. There are toilets with baby changing and a friendly café, selling hot and cold snacks, including bacon barms, toasties, cups of tea and hot vimto. Tables can be found inside and there's also an outdoor picnic area.

It is worth calling in for maps of the park and a History Trail booklet, as you can do short walks into the park or longer trails that link up other areas. There is also an orienteering course that is pushchair friendly. Despite being so close to the M60 the park is beautiful and diverse, with woodland, ponds, canals, rivers and a meadow. Most of the walkways from the visitor centre, although nice and flat, are along waterways which are all unguarded, so take care with young children. It is also only when you look over the edge of the path after about five minutes from the visitor centre that you realise you're actually on the old aqueduct 80 feet above the winding River Medlock.

In the summer, the river's a great spot for paddling. In June 2007, Lowry's 'Good Friday, Daisy Nook', sold at Christies for nearly £3.8 million, the highest price paid for the artist at auction. The Easter fair celebrated in this painting is still held at Daisy Nook every year.

Cafe: Mon-Fri 9.30am-4pm, Weekends 9am-5pm
Daisy Nook Country Park, Stannybrook Road, Failsworth, Manchester M35 9WJ
Tel: 0161 308 3909 www.oldhamparks.co.uk
Bus to: Oldham Road (396, 409, 419) Newmarket Road (168, 169, 230, 232, 233). Train to: Oldham or Ashton, then bus.

Etherow Country Park

With family staying for the weekend and feeling in the mood for a brisk country walk before lunch, we all headed to Etherow. One of Britain's first Country Parks, it's approximately 240 acres in the Etherow-Goyt Valley, rich with wildlife, fungi, waterways and plenty of child and pram friendly pathways. We set off from the pay and display car park in George Street, Compstall, situated by the visitor centre. Toilets and a café are also here. The visitor centre, which sells duck food, aims to be open daily 9am-5pm but they can't always man it so it's potluck.

TOP FIVE PARKS

Heaton Park
A vast, beautifully landscaped park. Go for tram rides, farm animals, land train and donkey rides.

Bruntwood Park
Fantastic set of three excellent playgrounds combined with ponds, wetlands and woodlands.

Chorlton Water Park
Ducks, geese, easy paths and a secret orchard make this one of our firm favourites.

Alderley Edge
Spectacular views, gorgeous woodlands and exciting climbs on fallen trees. A magical place.

Daisy Nook
Orienteering for pushchairs, ponds, canals, rivers and meadows. One of North Manchester's finest.

There were hundreds of birds by the man made lake at the start of the walk: pink-footed geese, swans and ducks amongst others, all ready to peck our fingers off. We took a pram friendly pathway that led past a small garden centre up the Goyt Valley alongside the waterway through woodland. We walked over and past a few footbridges perfect for Pooh Sticks. There were a couple of picnic tables overlooking the weir – a lovely place to eat on a summer's day. The circular walk to the weir and then round the lake took just over an hour and was very manageable for my 23 month old who didn't get in his stroller once. After our walk, we spent some time watching the sailing boats on the lake before having a quick cup of tea and juice in the cafe. High chairs and baby change facilities are both available.

Cafe: Daily 10am-4pm
Pay and display car park.
Etherow Country Park, Compstall, Stockport SK6 5HN
Tel:0161 427 6937
Bus to: Andrew Street (304/306, 383/384, 394). Train to: Romiley or Marple, then bus.

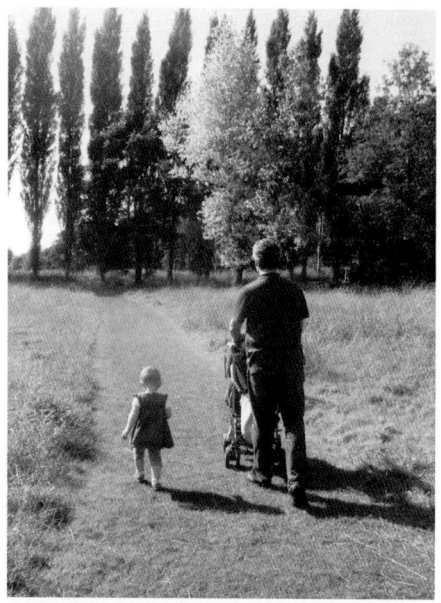

Grace with her Daddy in Fletcher Moss, a beautiful park in Didsbury, it is lovely at any time of year.

Parks, woods and walks

Heaton Park

One of the largest publicly owned parks in Europe (650 acres, Grade II listed) and just four miles north of the city centre, there is loads to see and do with little ones in beautiful Heaton Park. There are four car parks so look on a map before you go to work out which one's best.

First off we visited the Farm Centre – home to pigs, cows, sheep, rabbits and… alpacas! The animals were slightly upstaged by the tiny outside play area with its wooden tractor. Thankfully the lure of a donkey ride proved too much. The very cute donkeys from the farm are harnessed up most weekends to give children rides for £1 in a large meadow area at the front of the buildings – it was a huge success.

Next up was the land train (runs every day through summer and school holidays from 11am) which takes you on a generous circuit round the park for £2 each. It's perfect because Heaton Park isn't short on hills with its spectacular views over the Pennines, so the train gives you chance to rest your legs a bit. Obviously the kids love it – there's lots of toots and waving to passers by going on. They were very accommodating with prams as

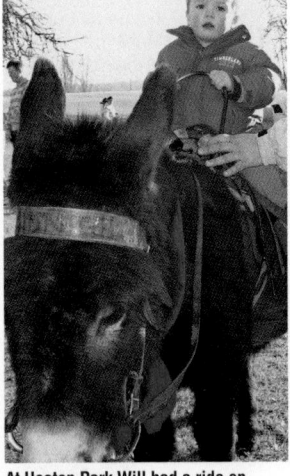

At Heaton Park Will had a ride on Midnight the donkey, rode the land train and visited the farm!

well – wait for the conductor (don't try and lift it in as we did!) – he'll point you in the direction of a couple of specially adapted carriages that have built in ramps so you can just push your buggy in and sit next to it.

There are two restaurants – The Stables near the farm and The Boathouse pavilion in a gorgeous setting right next to the lake. It's basically self-service though you can order a selection of hot platters – the food was ok. Highchairs available and baby changing in toilets. There are bottle warming facilities in the cafes. After lunch we hit the playgrounds – there are two large children's areas providing a range of activities for 3-14 year olds.

We'd run out of time by now but worth mentioning is that there are also rowing boats for hire daily, out of season it's weekends only, weather permitting. Cost is £8.50 for up to four people for 45 minutes.

Vintage tram rides operate on Sundays from Easter till the end of September (with limited winter opening times so best check first). When they're running, there is one

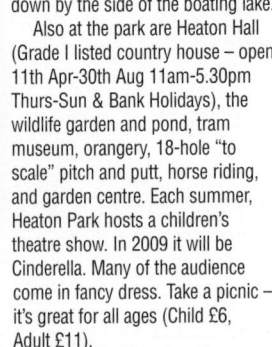

tram working at any given time, although you can look at the range of trams down at the depot. The tram experience is operated from here to just short of the lakeside on a small length of track (price may change but currently the all day ticket price is £2). During most school holidays you're also likely to find a fairground down by the side of the boating lake.

Also at the park are Heaton Hall (Grade I listed country house – open 11th Apr-30th Aug 11am-5.30pm Thurs-Sun & Bank Holidays), the wildlife garden and pond, tram museum, orangery, 18-hole "to scale" pitch and putt, horse riding, and garden centre. Each summer, Heaton Park hosts a children's theatre show. In 2009 it will be Cinderella. Many of the audience come in fancy dress. Take a picnic – it's great for all ages (Child £6, Adult £11).

If, like us, you're visiting the Farm Centre, the best car park to use is accessed on St Margaret's Road, off Bury Old Road. Car parking is £1 at weekends.

Animal Centre open daily Good Friday-Sept 10.30am-7pm (in school holidays) and 10.30am-5pm (during term time); Sept-Mar 10.30am-3.30pm
Heaton Park, Junction 18 or 19 of the M60, Off Middleton Road (A576), Prestwich, Manchester M25 2SW
Tel: 0161 773 1085 www.heatonpark.org.uk
Bus to: Bury Old Road (135, 137, 138, 495) or Middleton Road (59, 64, 115, 156, 164, 167). Tram to: Heaton Park.
Train to: Manchester city centre, then bus or tram.

Fletcher Moss Botanical Gardens

Fletcher Moss really is one of Manchester's gems. Whether in summer or winter, this park is beautiful. There is limited parking off Millgate Lane and on Stenner Lane, but beware of parking in the Didsbury Pub car park as there are clamping signs everywhere.

The café opens most weekends and daily through the summer months, as well as occasionally on a cold but bright winter's day. There is a small visitor centre at the bottom of the building behind the café which is open Mon-Fri 8am-4pm, but only at weekends if there is a warden. Toilets are always

open, but they have no baby changing facilities.

If you have managed to get past the café without being tempted by the cakes, the old bowling green is now a pergola garden with wooden arches and roses, making it an ideal picnic spot as dogs aren't allowed. There is a beautiful sloping botanical garden that follows a small stream down to a clay pond at the bottom. If you can keep the children quiet for long enough, you can see terrapins sunbathing on the lily pads.

My kids love this park for scootering as the gentle slopes make it a bit more exciting than other places, although they do tend to shatter the peace and tranquillity as they fly down the hill! You can continue on into Stenner Wood. Although often flooded in autumn, in spring it is full of bluebells and snowdrops. If you carry straight on you reach the River Mersey.

There is a paved path that leads back to Stenner Lane, and across the road you'll find Parsonage Gardens. This is a lovely spot with rare trees and beautiful gardens. It also contains the original orchid house that is open if the ranger is there. You'll find koi carp and goldfish in the pond inside.

Fletcher Moss Botanical Gardens, Wilmslow Road, Manchester M20 2SW Tel: 0161 434 1877
Bus to: Wilmslow Road (23, 23A, 42, 42A, 171, 196, 370, 195, 196, 142, X57). Train to: East Didsbury, then bus.

Haigh Hall and Country Park

Surrounded by over 250 acres of stunning park and woodland, Haigh Hall boasts magnificent panoramas as far reaching as north Wales. Start by popping in to the information and gift shop for a map and advice on the most pram-friendly walks. We enjoyed a very leisurely (translate: slow) stroll around with the pram and despite me being heavily pregnant and hence a tad immobile, the route we took was perfectly manageable. There are plenty of nature trails on offer for all levels of walking ability as well as the chance to explore the lovely woodlands steeped in flora and wildlife. We also saw tons of different varieties of birds around on our visit, which was wonderful. The Georgian Grade II listed hall is generally used for private functions although it is open to the public for events such as craft fairs. There's a playground with plenty of swings and a climbing frame but not much else. In season you'll also find a ladybird ride, bouncy castle and a miniature railway that takes you on a scenic ride around the woodlands. The train is open Easter-Sept weekends, school holidays and Sept-Easter (Sundays) weather permitting 1-4pm.

The café is open every day serving a selection of meals, snacks and drinks. Toilets with baby changing facilities. Pay and display car parking costs £1.50.

Haigh Country Park, Haigh, Wigan WN2 1PE Tel: 01942 832895 www.wlct.org/leisure/Haigh/ haighhome.ht

Holcombe Hill

As a child I lived for a time at the foot of Holcombe Hill and therefore I'm rather fond of it, or more particularly of Peel Tower perched at the top. It was built to commemorate Sir Robert Peel, former prime minister and founder of the modern police force. I have since returned with my children and we have enjoyed the spectacular views of Manchester and North Wales sat at the top of the hill eating a picnic.

On first assessment, there isn't anything child friendly about it; the paths are mainly inaccessible for pushchairs and there are no toilets or places to eat. I therefore wouldn't recommend it for people who would struggle carrying children some of the way. The hill however is an achievable walk for older toddlers and for parents carrying children in a papoose or back carrier. There is a village and pub close by offering refreshments and toilets, so for that reason I would recommend it as a place for a good family walk. Oliver, my three year old, certainly demonstrated a sense of achievement at reaching the top of the hill and after our picnic, enjoyed rolling back down parts of it again.

The tower is open on various days of the year, so if you can manage a further 150 steps after the hill climb, try and coincide your visit with an open day. On Good Friday morning it is traditional to roll eggs down the hill, and you will usually find children of all ages taking part.

Car parking available on Lumb Carr Road.

Holcombe Hill, Accessible from Lumb Carr Road Holcombe Village, Bury www.bury.gov.uk
Bus to: Bolton Road West. (273, 472, 473, 474, 475, 476, 477, 481, 485, X35). Tram to: Bury, then bus. Train to: Manchester, then bus or tram.

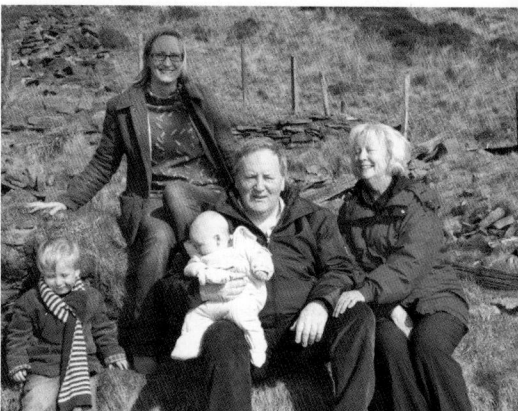

Holcombe Hill is an achievable walk for older toddlers and for parents carrying children in a papoose or back carrier. I would recommend it as a place for a good family walk and Ollie and Felix are pictured with Grandad and Granny Jean.

Hollingworth Lake Country Park

The two and a quarter mile flat perimeter path round Hollingworth Lake offers a superb walk if you have toddlers and pushchairs in tow. The lake is man made (dating back to 1800) but appears natural and has beautiful countryside surrounding it. On a clear autumn day I took my parents, a three year old and a baby. The three year old managed to walk almost the whole distance without stopping, and was kept entertained by muddy puddles, a bridge over a weir, plenty of wildlife (ducks to feed, birds, rabbits, domestic dogs), throwing pebbles in the lake (not at the wildlife) from the small beach, and if that was not enough there is a small children's playground at the end of our circular route. There were plenty of benches for grandparents who want to sit and take it in or eat a picnic. After our walk however we opted for fish and chips from a shop at the side of the lake.

Pay and display parking is available at the visitors centre on Rakewood Road where there is also a cafe, toilets and the children's playground. In the summer, rowing boats are available for hire and there is a ferry service across the lake. There is also a vast network of paths and woodland, not suitable for pushchairs, which connect to the perimeter walk. These are great for toddlers who are good at walking or if you are using a papoose. A couple of pleasant pubs overlook Hollingworth Lake. I understand they offer meals and bar snacks, making it an attractive choice for a Sunday walk followed by a pub lunch.

Baby change in disabled toilet.

Visitor centre Daily Apr-Oct 9.30am-5pm, Nov-Mar Mon-Fri 11am-4pm, Weekends 10.30am-5pm
Café Daily Apr-Oct 10am-4pm, Nov-Mar Mon-Fri 11.30am-3.30pm, Weekends 11am-4pm
Alice Ferry: weather permitting Apr-Oct Weekends 1-5pm, school summer holidays Mon-Sun 1-5pm
Crossing: Adult £1.50, Child £1
Circle of Lake: Adult £2.50, Child £1.50
Rowing Boats: weather permitting Apr-Oct all day but no life preserves available.
Hollingworth Lake, Rakewood Road, Littleborough, Rochdale OL15 0AQ
Tel: 01706 373421 www.rochdale.gov.uk
Bus to: Lake Bank (452, 455, 456). Train to: Smithy Bridge, then walk.

Moses Gate Country Park

Restored from an old industrial site, the beautiful 305 hectare park is a place of national scientific interest due to its unique wildlife. It's easy to find and there's plenty of free parking – we parked at the bottom car-park which brings you virtually straight into the excellent children's play ground and the Rock Hall Visitor Centre. Moses Gate is centred on three lakes with miles of scenic parkland to take a walk in. There are pathways and seating round the lakes and the area we ambled round was nice and flat so access with a pram is easy. There's no café (a couple of burger vans at the entrance) but plenty of well-maintained picnic areas. There are lots of fun sounding "Toddler Walks" with the ranger each month aimed at pre-school children and their families, so phone ahead to find out what's coming up.

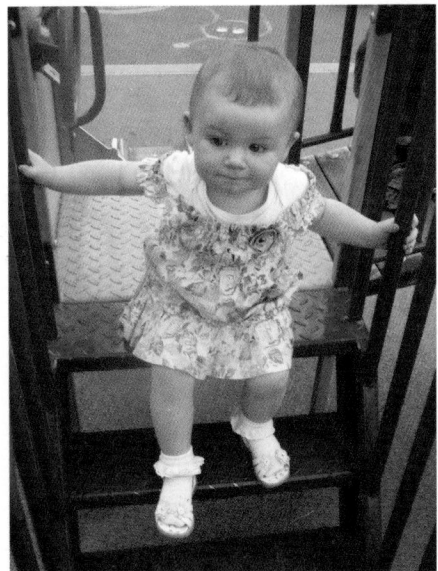

With two playgrounds, Platt Fields is a very good town centre park. Grace loves the climbing frame.

Visitor centre Mon-Sun 9.30am-4.30pm (Baby changing in the visitor centre toilets).
Moses Gate Country Park, Rock Hall Visitor Centre, Hall Lane, Farnworth, Bolton, BL4 7QN
Tel: 01204 334343 www.bolton.gov.uk
Bus to: Bolton Road (8, 22, 37, 512, 513, 521, 534, 556).
Train to: Moses Gate.

Moss Bank Park

In the summer holidays Moss Bank Park has an assortment of fun fair rides and activities, including a bouncy castle, an enormous inflatable slide and a carousel. In winter it is much more sedate park, which is how I prefer it.

Moss Bank Park is also home to Animal World, which sounds quite grand and raises your expectations. Grand it isn't, but this is a free attraction and it is definitely worth a visit. You enter via the Butterfly House that is actually pretty good, with wooden walkways over a running stream where you can see lots of fish, and butterflies are flying overhead in the tropical environment. You then move outside to a selection of animals and birds with peacocks roaming freely, as well as guinea pigs and farm animals, plus some very cute chipmunks.

The play area is comprehensive, with large slides and climbing frames and two huge sandpits. In the summer it can get busy at weekends. There is also a miniature steam railway running on Sundays throughout the year, weather permitting. It is run by a fantastic team of volunteers who do try and operate more frequently during the summer.

Parking is free. Park in the bottom main car park as the small one at the top is for blue badge holders only. There are toilets in the car park but they tend to be open only in summer. The toilets by Animal World are always open but unfortunately there are no baby changing facilities in either block.

There is a small café (open during the sumer and at weekends in winter) doing a great trade in tea and ice creams, but what I liked was the Hot Vimto for £1 – being a typical southerner, honestly, I'd never heard of it! Something I'm still taking stick for. Unfortunately they can't warm up baby bottles.

Animal World Open: 1st Apr-30th Sep Mon-Sun 10am-4.30pm, 1st Oct-31st Mar Mon-Thur 10am-3.30pm, Fri 10am-2.30pm, Weekends 10am-3.30pm
Animal World and Butterfly House, Moss Bank Park, Moss Bank Way, Bolton BL1 6NQ
Animal World Tel: 01204 334050
Moss Bank Park Tel: 01204 334121
www.bolton.org.uk/mossbank.html
Bus to: Lightbounds Road (519) Church Road (501).
Train to: Bolton, then bus.

Philips Park

Opened in 1846, Philips Park is one of the world's first municipal parks. It's still crammed with original features including the carriage drive, serpentine paths and plantation although its Victorian splendour has worn a little thin. It's situated next to the City of Manchester Stadium and covers 31 acres with the River Medlock running through the middle. We found the best place to leave the car was on Stuart Street – the entrance there brings you straight in at the younger children's play area, then you can drop down towards the duck pond and have more of a walk round the bottom area of the park if you wish. It's all very accessible with plenty of footpaths and not overly steep. Toilets are in the lodge at the entrance close to the playground (open approx same hours as park however less likely to be open at weekends because the warden is often not available).

Philips Park, Stuart Street, Manchester M11 4DQ
Tel: 0161 231 3090 www.philipspark.org.uk
Bus to: Alan Turing Way (53, 54, 185, 217, 218) Briscoe Lane (74, 76, 77, 78 113). Train to: Ashburys, then bus (53).

Platt Fields Park

Although not the prettiest, Platt Fields has a lot to offer. There are two great playgrounds for small children, one specifically for under 5s with lots of age appropriate equipment and a central boating lake which is paved all round. During the summer you can hire boats for around £5 for half an hour

for up to four people. Through the rest of the park there are walking paths where you tend to stumble on some rather nice little mini-gardens such as the Shakespearean garden and the Eco Arts Garden which is great for exploring.

Toilets are in the Lakeside Centre with baby changing in the disabled toilet, open every day. If you're driving, the car park isn't signposted and it's tucked down off Mabfield Road with a one way system in operation.

Platt Fields Park, Wilmslow Road, Fallowfield, Manchester M14 6LA
Tel: 0161 224 2902 www.plattfields.org
Bus to: Wilmslow Road (41, 42, 42A, 43, 44, 46/47, 48, 111, 142, 143, X57). Train to: Manchester city centre or East Didsbury, then bus.

Reddish Vale Country Park

Reddish Vale Country Park is over 398 acres of green belt along the River Tame in the heart of Stockport. Depending on where you think you might end up, you can either park at the bottom of the hill by the country park and walk up to Reddish Vale Farm and tea rooms or park by the farm and walk down to the country park. Either way parking is free and is less than a five minute walk.

To your left as you come to the bottom of the hill there is a little mill pond with great views of the viaduct and The Vale. To your right, past a small visitor centre there is a wooded area heading down to another pond with a large wooden walkway enclosed by the river. There is also a large grassy area surrounded by a paved walk which is the butterfly conservation park.

There are no baby changing facilities in the toilets by the visitor centre but some are available at Reddish Vale Farm – (see page 34).

Tearooms: Sat 9am-4pm, Sun 9.30am-4pm. Open daily in school holidays 9.30am-4pm. Tel: 0161 480 1645
Visitor Centre: Weekends, school holidays and bank/holidays 11am-4.30pm
Reddish Vale Country Park, Mill Lane, end of Reddish Vale Road, Reddish, Stockport, SK5 7HE
Tel: 0161 477 5637
www.reddishvale.moonfruit.com

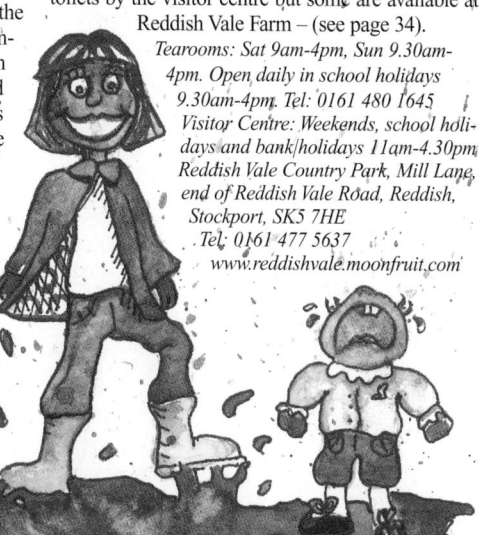

Parks, woods and walks

Sale Water Park and Broad Ees Dole Nature Reserve

The Mersey Valley is an important wildlife corridor running through the urban areas of Manchester and Trafford. It's a huge sector made up of wetlands, grasslands and woodlands. Our walk started at the Mersey Valley Visitor Centre where we parked the car. It's probably worth calling in and picking up a couple of free maps to give you a sense of the region. We visited in October but apparently the bank of wildflowers below the visitor centre is awash with colour during summer months and a good place to spot butterflies.

We set off down a pathway in the direction of Broad Ees Dole Nature Reserve walking alongside Sale Water Park. The footpath was gentle and well surfaced and for the most part quite protected by tree canopies with gaps exposing views of the marshland and of course the lake. Despite it being a blustery day our three year old walked about a mile, which took us just into the Nature Reserve. Broad Ees Dole was formerly a flood meadow – the area now incorporates wetland, reed beds, meadow and woodland habitats. There are no footpaths leading through the Dole, they are around the perimeter and provide excellent viewpoints to watch the birds.

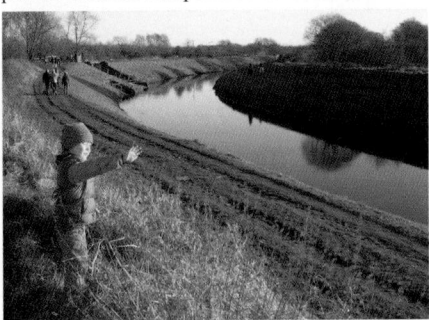

A family walk along the Mersey River linking Sale and Chorlton Water Park.

We headed back towards the car and decided to take refuge in Café Ark which is adjacent to the visitor centre. It's a great little find, quite small – only six tables inside but several outside if weather fine. It's nicely individual, with paintings hanging on the wall, books and magazines to browse through and wonderful smells wafting out of the kitchen. There's a large blackboard just underneath the serving counter and children are invited to draw. We didn't eat but the food, all vegetarian and all made from scratch, looked great – lasagne was £4.95, cheese on toast was £2.50 and omelettes £3.50 amongst lots of other tempting dishes. Happy to provide water to heat up bottles and will blend any food for baby. Several high chairs available.

Toilets are located opposite the car-park and are open seven days a week 10am-4pm. Baby changing is due to be fitted into the disabled toilet and should be available 2009.

Café Ark: Winter Weds-Sun 11am-4pm,
Summer Weds-Sun and Bank Holidays 11am-5pm
Tel: 0161 969 6775
Visitors Centre: Winter Tues-Fri 11am-4pm, weekends 1-4pm, Summer Tues-Fri 11am-5pm, weekends 1.30-5pm
Mersey Valley Visitor Centre, Rifle Road, Sale Water Park, Sale, Cheshire M33 2LX
Tel: 0161 905 1100   www.merseyvalley.org.uk
Bus to: Chorlton Bus Station (22, 23, 23A, 46, 47, 84, 85, 86, 168, 270, 279). Tram to: Manchester city centre or Altrincham Interchange, then bus. Train to: Manchester city centre or Altrincham, then bus.

Vernon Park

Vernon Park is Stockport's oldest park, opened in 1858. It's a grand old place, typical of Victorian civic parks. Restored to its former glory in 2000 after decades of neglect, it's a beautiful open space overlooking the Goyt Valley and its river below.

In truth there's not a lot here designed for small children. There's no playground, nor any bespoke facilities. Not only that but Vernon Park is built in to a steep hill and walking up with toddler and buggy is not for the faint hearted (though heading back down on a micro scooter delighted our little boy whilst exhausting his protective dad). But, for all of its child-friendly flaws, this is a glorious park. There are lawns and fountains and cannons and sculpture and even a maze; all of which provided us with plenty of fun.

There's also a small café and slightly idiosyncratic (but miniscule) museum containing artefacts of Stockport history with some Egyptian mummies thrown in for good measure. There is no lift access however. The café and terrace were good for a cuppa and a light snack and they will heat up baby bottles etc. Toys were provided together with a few children's chairs and a little table. Both café and museum are run by Pure Innovations (a not for profit charity) and felt like a labour of love. A Tots group runs every Thurs 10am-12noon (£2) – phone ahead to book in. Baby changing in the ladies toilets downstairs.

Café and museum open weekdays 10am-4pm; weekends 11am-4pm (Bank Holidays and April-Sep until 5pm).
Vernon Park, Turncroft Lane, Stockport SK1 4AR
Tel: 0161 474 4460 www.stockport.gov.uk
Bus to: 330, 380/381, 383/384, 389. Train to: Stockport, then bus.

Wythenshawe Park

This public park covering around 250 acres in south Manchester has got a lot to offer – a working community farm, a play ground, a sixteenth century hall and even a horticultural centre. The parkland's

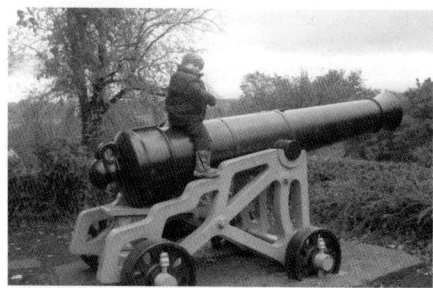

WIll was happy with the cannons and fountains at Vernon Park. Built into a steep hill it's not for the faint-hearted.

got historic and ornamental woodlands to explore, formal flowerbeds to admire and beautiful wildflower meadows.

Visit the glasshouses and you'll find yourself pointed in the direction of the Safari walk which takes you from cacti terrain through to a rainforest section: the Jungle walk – a massively overgrown area with a couple of ponds with fish and then outside lots of herbs to smell and touch. It's all via little pathways and bridges which the children like. There's even an aviary!

The small farm (a registered charity) is always our main reason to visit. Because it's free and on our doorstep, it feels easy just to pop in for half an hour. There are cows, sheep, pigs, horses and chickens – the usual suspects. You can usually buy eggs here as well, which the children enjoy. If you're after a pleasant walk, a trip to a playground and a few animals, then Wythenshawe Park's definitely worth a look.

The Courtyard Tea Rooms are a relatively new addition located in the historic stables just behind the hall. It was extremely friendly when we went. Although the menu's quite short, it's reasonably priced and we enjoyed our sandwiches and soup just fine. There are high chairs and the staff will provide hot water for baby bottles. Baby changing is in the disabled toilets and they're open daily 9am-4.30pm.

£1 Car park charges apply only Apr-Nov weekends and Bank Holidays.
Farm: Daily 11.30am-3.30pm;
Glass Houses: Daily 10am-4pm (weather dependant)
Courtyard Tea Rooms: weekends 10am-5pm and daily through school holidays.
Hall: April-Sept, weekends 10am-5pm
Wythenshawe Park, Wythenshawe Road, Manchester M23 0AB Tel: 0161 998 2117 www.manchestergov.uk Bus to: Altrincham Road (99,101, 179, 264, 371) or Wythenshawe Road (370). Tram to: Altrincham Interchange, then bus. Train to: Altrincham, then bus.

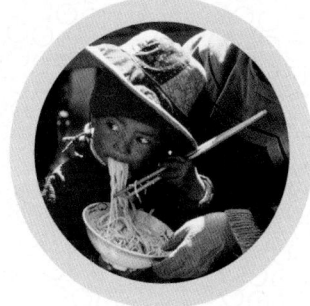
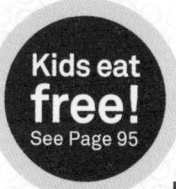

OUT AND ABOUT

Planes, trains and automobiles

As you'd expect from the cradle of the industrial revolution, Manchester is one great big opportunity to express your love of moving vehicles of every type. And let's face it, which small child doesn't thrill to a plane, a train or a Victorian hydraulic boat lift? They're all here and a lot more besides.

Planes, trains and automobiles

PLANES

Aviation Viewing Park

As we went to press the Aviation Viewing Park was undergoing a massive overhaul costing more than £1 million. Replacing the static burger van and basic but clean toilet facilities will be a huge hangar to house Concorde as well as provide a restaurant, toilets and a new shop. There will also be a smaller hangar to accommodate a visitors' centre and modest museum. Another addition will be an educational suite that will replicate the experience you have at the airport when you go on holiday. Unfortunately this element will only be on offer to groups, but that will include toddler groups.

Currently though, and this will remain the same during the overhaul, you will find three raised viewing mounds offering great views of both take-off and landing aircraft. There is also a Monarch and DC-10 but these can only be viewed from the outside or as part of an organised tour. The Trident and the AVRO RJX are both available to have a look round at weekends for £1.50 but they are probably more suited to older children.

In terms of parking, there is ample space but it is always busy so be careful with toddlers running around. There are large grassy areas and picnic tables available if you want to bring some lunch.
Mon-Sun 8.30am till dusk. Admission currently £4 per car including driver and £1 for every passenger or pedestrian, under 5s free.
Aviation Viewing Park, Sunbank Lane, Altrincham WA15 8XQ Tel: 0161 489 3932
www.manchesterairport.co.uk
Bus to: Wilmslow Old Road terminus (200). Train to: Manchester Airport.

Concorde moving in to its new £1 million hangar at the Aviation Viewing Park.

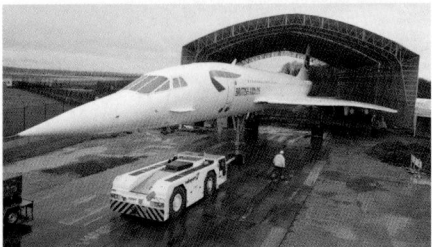

The Airport Hotel

I'd heard about the Airport Hotel but my visit definitely exceeded expectations. Admittedly from the front it looks rather like an unassuming pub, but the rear sits just 50 feet from the final approach for Manchester Airport's Runway 23R, and the close-up views of aircraft landing are superb.

The car park at the pub is a small pay and display, but for £3 for one hour you get a £2 voucher redeemable against food or drink purchased inside; £5 for up to four hours' parking entitles you to a £4 voucher. Do not park on the road as you're likely to end up with a £60 parking ticket.

Once in the pub, head out the back through the sliding doors. You'll find an enormous, safely enclosed beer garden with plenty of picnic tables and despite it being a windy, overcast day when we were there, Harry and Sam loved the wooden climbing frame. There are also a few ride-on machines so it is an idea to have some change ready. During the summer holidays, and weather permitting, there is a bouncy castle and barbecue at weekends.

Planes land from your left-hand side, but quite often, depending on the wind, aircraft use the holding point on your right-hand side for take-off and the noise is tremendous.

The pub does a children's menu for £2.50 for fishfingers/burgers/nuggets and chips but it also includes a tomato and pasta option so is a little more varied than the 'everything with chips' first impression. And you can get a nice pint of real ale so it's not all for the kids. There is a dedicated family room open until 9pm. Baby changing facilities are in the ladies' toilet.
Mon-Sun 7.30am-9pm admission free.
The Airport Hotel, Ringway Road, Manchester M22 5WH Tel: 0161 437 2551
www.theairporthotel.com
Bus to: Ringway Road (19, 200, 369). Train to: Manchester Airport, then bus.

TRAINS

Abbotsfield Park Miniature Railway

Abbotsfield Park in Flixton looks at first sight like any other small park. It's a recreation ground the size of a couple of football pitches with a small children's play area. However, just as you're crossing the bridge to the entrance you're drawn to a

Planes, trains and automobiles

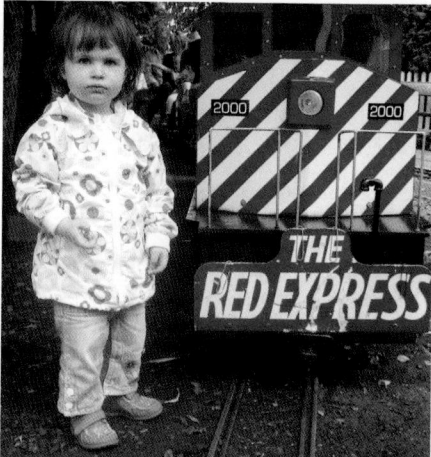

Clodagh at Brookside's authentic replica station, which has five locomotives – three steam engines and two diesel.

plume of steam coming towards you at some speed. This is the Abbotsfield Park Miniature Railway and miniature is the word. It's the smallest locomotive you've ever seen outside of a domestic train set. Our son watched rapt as this tiny engine thundered past with half-a-dozen people in tow. He couldn't wait to get on and do a couple of circuits of the park himself.

Arriving at the station, we discovered it was the HQ of the Urmston and District Model Engineering Society. The station stood next to the children's playground and an ice cream van was doing a roaring trade. This little railway is an absolute labour of love. It's been staffed by club members bringing delight to children since the late forties and is a local treasure. One to warm your heart.
Weather permitting, trains run Sundays and Bank Holidays from 11am-3.30pm in winter and 11am-4.30pm in summer. There is occasional opening on Wednesdays too during school holidays.
Rides are 20p per person.
Abbotsfield Park and Urmston & District Model Engineering Society, Chassen Rd, Flixton, Manchester M41 5DH Tel: 0161 748 0160
http://homepages.tesco.net/david.a.roberts
Bus to: Flixton Road (255, 268) or Church Road (243, 253, 276, 278). Train to: Chassen Road.

Brookside Miniature Railway

We always have a fun time here – I can't get Will or his Daddy away from it! Brookside, located at a garden centre, has five locomotives – three steam engines and two diesel. The trains are located at their very own station, Brookside Central, which is a replica West Country station with authentic buildings, sidings, turntable and original signage on the miniature platform.

Inside the waiting room (which doubles as a gift shop and museum), you purchase your ticket then it's all aboard! The train takes you on a half-mile circuit through tunnels (one of which is 65ft long), over streams and level crossings and around the perimeter of the centre. It costs £1.30 per person (free for under 2s) and lasts about eight minutes.

After several goes on the train we usually end up at the little children's play area, where there's a life-size static tank engine that you can climb a ladder and have a look at as well as several ride-on machines – Postman Pat, Thomas the Tank Engine and a kiddie tramway (where the children ride along a short track by themselves). Also on site is a children's pottery studio where you can paint your own pots. During summer months and school holidays you'll often find a small children's funfair at one end of the garden centre, which the train chugs round and makes a stop at for anyone wanting a quick game of hook-a-duck.

Food wise there's two choices – a small coffee shop or the larger Romany Restaurant, which does have a children's menu available.

Baby changing is in the disabled toilets in the main garden centre.

Brookside offers children's railway parties for those mad about trains, which is ideal as a novel birthday theme.
Weekends all year round 11am-4pm, also in addition Weds April-Sept and school and Bank Holidays. Closed Easter Sunday. Steam locomotives only run duringweekends.
Brookside Garden Centre, Macclesfield Road (A523), Poynton, Cheshire SK12 1BY Tel: 01625 875756
www.brooksidegardencentre.com
Bus to: Fiveways (307/308, 108, 191, 390, 392, 393).
Train to: Hazel Grove, then bus.

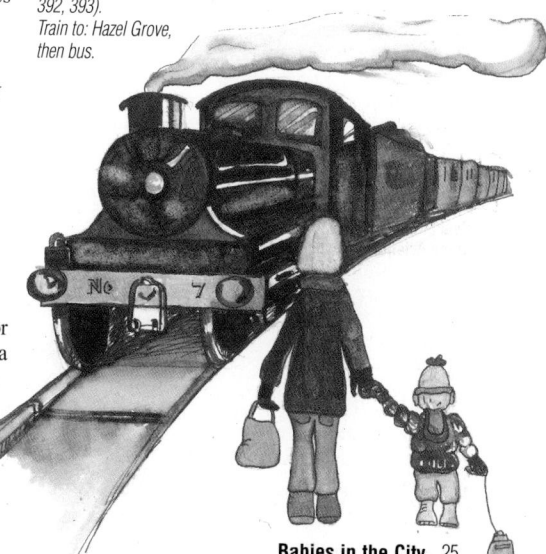

Planes, trains and automobiles

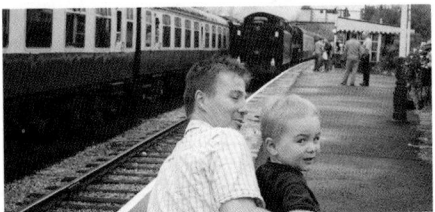

Arriving at Bury's Bolton Street Station is like stepping back in time.

East Lancashire Railway

Arriving at Bury's Bolton Street Station is like stepping back in time. There are traditional ticket booths, lovely signage and helpful staff.

We decided to go from Bury to Ramsbottom but for a longer ride you can take the train from Heywood all the way to Rawtenstall. There is a pay and display car park at Bury Station Mon-Fri which is free at weekends, but be careful as other Bury car parks charge on a Saturday.

At Bury Station The Trackside pub, situated on Platform 2, does children's meals at £2.25 for sausage or fishfingers with chips and beans, and they are happy to warm up bottles or baby food. Baby changing is in the disabled toilets at the end of Platform 2, there are also facilities at Ramsbottom Station. There are steps at Bury but staff are happy to help with pushchairs. Alternatively there is access to the platform by The Trackside and staff will accompany you across the track.

Ramsbottom is a 15-minute journey through some gorgeous Lancashire countryside. We've travelled on both diesel and steam trains and both are good, but I think the romance of the steam train wins. The boys loved it and had their heads pressed against the window for the entire journey. There is a buffet car on board as well as toilets. Ramsbottom station is only a five-minute walk away from shops and cafés and there are plenty of picnic tables by the station, as well as a children's park. A traditional country market can be found every Saturday and on the second Sunday of each month a farmers' market.

Family days run throughout the year and there are Santa Specials in December but pre-booking is essential. Bury Transport Museum is also due to re-open in September 2009 after a £3 million refurbishment.

Winter Weekends 3rd Jan-5th Apr, 19th Sep-27th Dec;
Summer Wed-Sun 8th Apr-13th Sep, plus bank holidays;
Santa Specials 22nd-24th Dec and weekends in December.
The Trackside, food available Mon-Thurs 12-3pm, Fri 12-6pm, Sat 9am-5pm, Sun 10am-5pm.
Return fares from Bury to Ramsbottom: Adult £6.60, Child £4.40, Under 5s free.
Bolton Street Station, Bolton Street, Bury, Lancashire BL9 0EY Tel: 0161 764 7790 www.east-lancs-rly.co.uk
Bus to: Bury Interchange. Tram to: Bury Interchange.
Train to: Manchester city centre, then bus or tram.

Dragon Miniature Railway

The Dragon Miniature Railway is located at a garden centre in Marple. There, just by the side of the car park, you'll find a little station with two trains (one diesel and one steam) running alternately on a half-mile track. For 70p each you'll be taken through a tunnel, alongside a river, via eccentric displays of garden gnomes and blow-up dinosaurs – you'll even get the chance to stop off at a small picnic and children's play area filled with Little Tikes style toys – open Mar-Oct.

The railway is run by enthusiasts and is a nice way to while away some time before popping into the garden centre for a mooch around the bedding plants. There's a selection of 20p ride-on machines next to the train station and also 'Tara the Tram', a little tram that self-propels up a short track where you can even ring a bell – all very sweet!

The garden centre itself has a fairly substantial café that offers a children's menu.

Weekends and school holidays (weather dependent) 11am-4.30pm.
Dragon Miniature Railway, Wyevale Garden Centre, Otherspool, Dooley Lane, Marple, Stockport SK6 7HE
Tel: 0774 8581160
Bus to: Stockport Road (358, 383/384), then walk.
Train to: Hazel Grove, then bus.

Hills Miniature Railway

Run by South Stockport Model Engineering Society, this delightful railway can be found at Hills Garden Centre, just south of Knutsford. There's an authentic station shop where you collect your £1 ticket (this doubles up as a gift shop selling toy

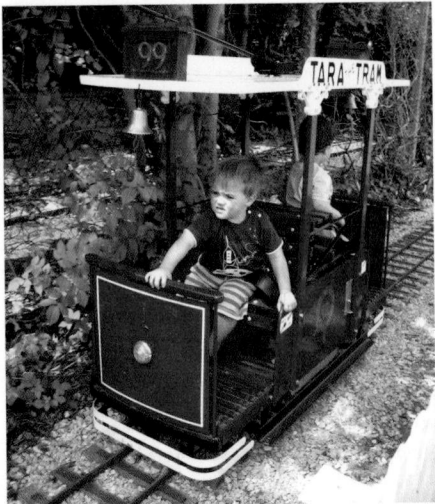

The Dragon Miniature Railway is run by enthusiasts. It has diesel and steam trains and a little tram that self-propels up a short track where you can ring a bell.

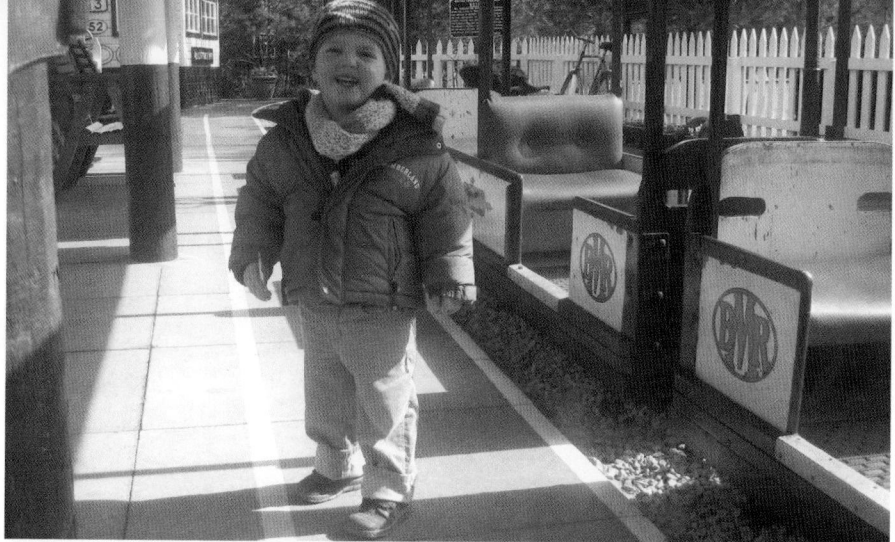

Hills Miniature Railway is a gem – if you've got a child like Will who's fanatical about trains, it's definitely worth a visit.

trains and accessories) and the train puffs its way around the perimeter of the garden centre, taking in the odd tunnel along the way.

Also at Hills is a Toby Tram – a self-drive tram popular with younger children, and a nine-hole miniature golf course. There's a lovely café but it does get busy and isn't very big so get there early if you're intending to have lunch. A good selection of hot and cold food is on offer and there is a dedicated children's menu as well. Probably worth mentioning: if you've got a child who's fanatical about trains, Hills does offer private railway parties.
Sun Jan-Easter, Weekends Easter-Sep, Sun Sep-Oct, closed Nov, weekend Santa specials in Dec 11am-4pm (weather dependent).
Hills Garden Centre, London Road, Allostock, Knutsford, Cheshire WA16 9LU
Tel: 07760 373466 www.hillsgardencentre.com

CABLE CAR AND BIG WHEEL

The Heights of Abraham

If you fancy a trip in a cable car… well, it's not impossible, but it's a bit of a drive. An hour and a half south in fact, through the Peak District to Matlock Bath in Derbyshire. If it does take your fancy, it's a good trip, as it's through stunning countryside, taking in the likes of Buxton, Bakewell (try a tart – nothing like the shop-bought ones) and Chatsworth.

The Heights of Abraham was Britain's first alpine style cable car when it opened in 1984. It's now a beautiful trip up over the Derwent Valley to Hilltop Park at the Heights. Once up there, as well as the fantastic views that have been enjoyed for centuries, you'll find caverns, woodlands, adventure playgrounds, a fossil factory, an amphitheatre which

hosts special events and a café. All told, a lovely way to while away a few hours on a clear day.
Mon-Sun 14th-22nd Feb 10am-4.30pm;
Weekends 28th Feb-21st March 10am-4.30pm;
Mon-Sun 21st March-1st Nov 10am-5pm.
Admission: Adult £10.80, Under 16s £7.80, Under 5s free. Family ticket £33.
The Heights of Abraham, Matlock Bath, Derbyshire DE4 3PD Tel: 01629 582365
www.heightsofabraham.com
Train to: Derby then on to Matlock Bath.

The Wheel of Manchester

On a recent trip into town we succumbed to the demands of our four-year-old and took a spin on The Wheel, Manchester's answer to the London Eye. For the time being The Wheel looks set to stay in Manchester and I for one think it's a very attractive addition to the city's landmarks.

There are 42 glass-panelled capsules to choose from and as it wasn't busy we didn't have to wait. We couldn't take the pushchair onboard, but they were happy for us to leave it at the bottom (although this is at your own risk).

The wheel gently rotates to reach a height of 60m, and if children start moving around to look on the other side, the pod does get a bit rocky. We went on a reasonably nice day and so were able to look out beyond the city centre to the surrounding countryside. It was interesting to have such a different perspective of this rapidly-changing city and to see landmarks such as Old Trafford, Urbis and Manchester Town Hall from above but I have to admit that by the third revolution the children were losing interest. That said, it's something different to do and the city skyline is definitely richer for having The Wheel as a key feature.

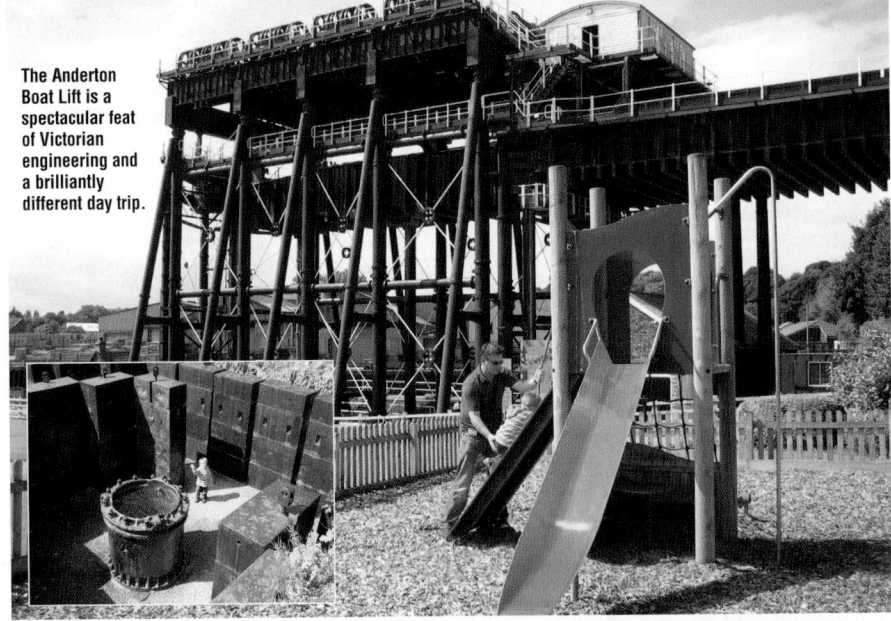

The Anderton Boat Lift is a spectacular feat of Victorian engineering and a brilliantly different day trip.

Sun-Thurs 10am-11pm, Fri 10am-midnight,
Sat 9am-midnight.
Admission: Adult £6.50, Child 4-12yrs £4.50,
1-3yrs £1, Under 1s free, Family ticket £20 (book
online for a 10% discount).
The Wheel of Manchester, Exchange Square,
Manchester Tel: 0161 831 9918
www.worldtouristattractions.co.uk
Bus to: Manchester city centre. Tram to: Manchester city centre
(nearest: Victoria). Train to: Manchester city centre (nearest: Victoria).

BOATS

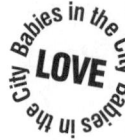
Babies in the City LOVE

Anderton Boat Lift

The Anderton Boat Lift in Cheshire is a spectacular feat of Victorian engineering and was the first of its kind in the world when it was built in 1875. It's a 50-foot vertical link between two waterways – the River Weaver and the Trent and Mersey Canal. It's hard to describe and do it justice so take a look at the picture!

For us it was a brilliantly different day trip. There are several admission options available. You can choose a lift trip – where you sit on a large glass-topped boat that sails from its mooring into the lift cradle and you either go from top to bottom or vice versa. Alternatively you can take a river trip – a gentle one-hour cruise in the same glass-topped boat. You can also combine the two, or merely visit the indoor exhibition.

We've got a fidgety two-and-a-half year old so we opted for the 35-minute lift trip. To be honest he got a bit restless even with that but it was worth it because it's such a lovely experience. Don't expect

an Alton Towers style ride though – it's very slow – in fact you hardly notice you're moving.

We had an hour's wait but there's a good visitor centre on site (complete with gift shop and café) and the exhibition has a few children's activities such as a drawing table and dressing up area. The café is pretty basic with standard fare such as jacket potatoes, sandwiches and children's lunchboxes (£2.75). Baby changing is in the ladies' toilets on the top floor and in the unisex downstairs in the exhibition.

Outside there's a small park, a maze and a water toy structure called 'canal adventure.' This consists of four plastic loops filled with water where you push your boat along and into little lifts (you need to hire a boat for 50p from the shop to play on this). There are also a couple of picnic areas with great views of the lift and river. The whole site is pushchair friendly – you can even take them on the boats with you (maximum of two allowed per trip).

In addition, if a family walk appeals, there's a large nature park next to the Boat Lift. The car park's located between the park and lift, but you do have to pay (£3 for all day).

Lift trip: Adult £7, Child £5; combined lift and river
trip: Adult £11, Child £8. Under 5s free.
Thurs-Sun 5th Feb-27th Mar and 5th-25th Nov,
11am-4pm, with no boat trip. Mon-Sun 28th Mar-4th
Oct 10am-5pm (Bank Holiday weekends until 6pm).
Lift trips start at 11am. Weds-Sun 7th Oct-1st Nov
11am-4pm. Lift trips start at 11.30am. Closed in Dec.
Anderton Boat Lift, Lift Lane, Anderton, Northwich,
Cheshire CW9 6FW Tel: 01606 786777
www.andertonboatlift.co.uk
Bus to: Anderton. Train to: Northwich.

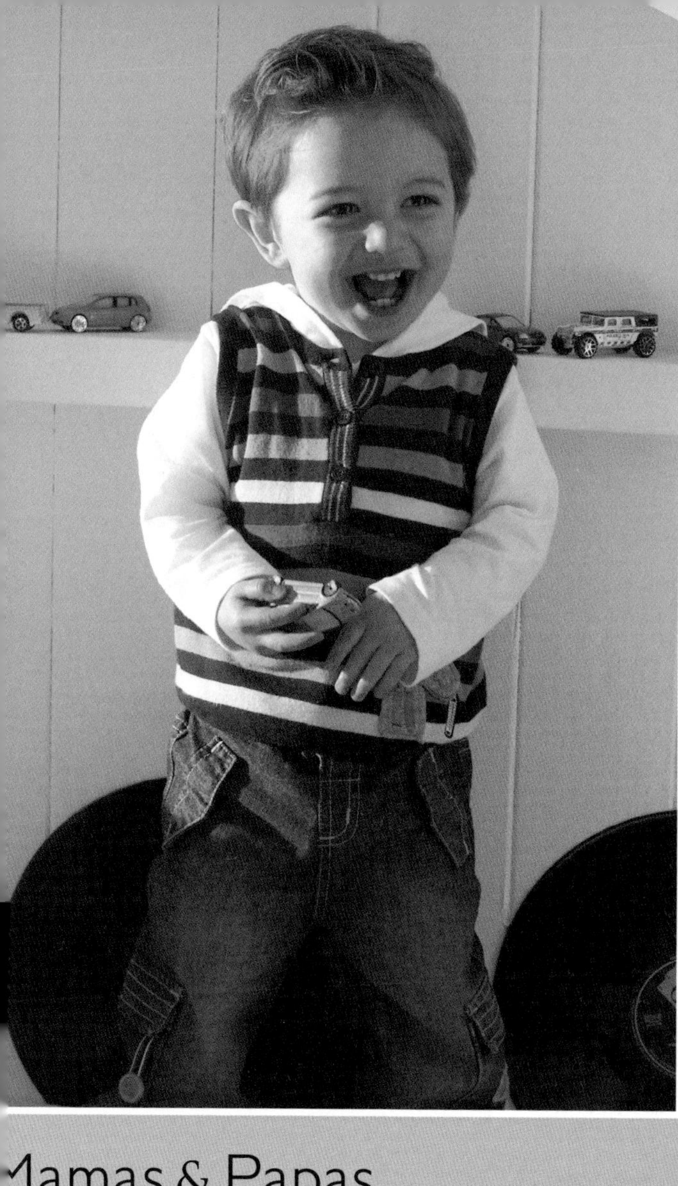

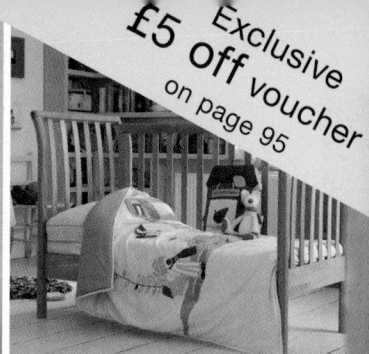

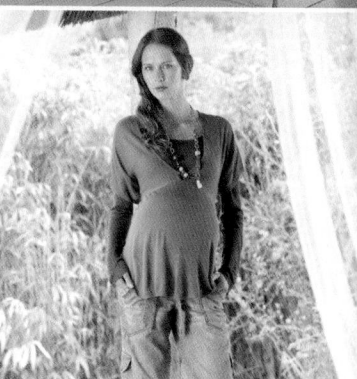

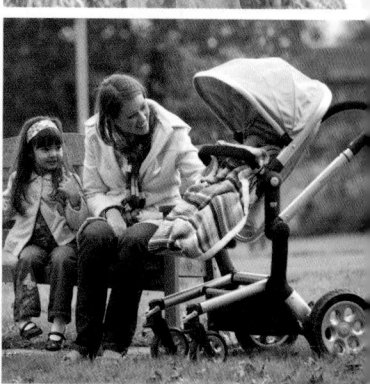

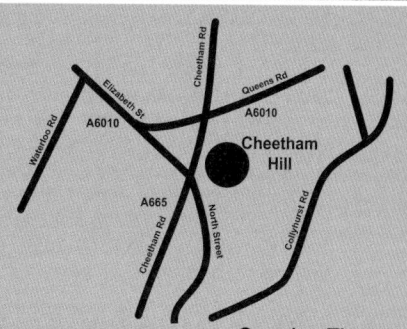

Mamas & Papas

Manchester Fort Shopping Park

Mamas & Papas
Manchester Fort Shopping Park
Cheetham Hill Road
Manchester,
8 8EP
mamasandpapas.com

Opening Times
Monday - Friday   10.00 - 20.00
Saturday   09.00 - 18.00
Sunday   11.00 - 17.00

Animals, nature and wildlife

You may be living in a city but you'll find creatures of all shapes and sizes to delight or terrify little ones not too far away.

Animals, nature and wildlife

Blue Planet Aquarium

I went with a group of mums plus kids on a typical rainy day. It is free entry for children under 95cm (around 2 and a half years old) otherwise a child price is £10.50 which I feel is quite steep and buying a family ticket only saves £2. The queue at the entrance was long but it did move fairly quickly. On bank holidays it would be wise to book ahead and fast track the queue.

It is a big aquarium, laid out over two floors with the majority being below ground. There is lift access to both floors but this is quite small although it's meant to take four pushchairs. The centre piece to Blue Planet is the fantastic Aquatunnel – 70 metres of underwater tunnels with sharks and manta rays floating only inches away. I lost count of how many times we went through the tunnel, until I realised the children had become more enthralled with the moving walkway! On busy days this section can be a nightmare with a pushchair. Half way round the tunnel section in a separate 2,000 litre tank is the Caribbean reef; this is where the children at last get to see lots of Nemos!

The aquatheatre, a partially seated auditorium with a massive picture window into the aquarium gives you a sense of just how large these sharks really are. There is a regular show where divers get in to feed the fish.

All the children enjoyed the rock pools where you can stroke the rays. There aren't many who don't relish the opportunity of getting wet! This area does get very busy and you have to wait for someone to get bored so you can squeeze in. Washbasins are around to wash your hands in after. The café area is large but very tightly packed with tables so it's difficult to manoeuvre your pushchair. Set out in a fast food chain style they offer hot and cold meal deals such as chicken nuggets and chips, a drink and fruit for around £3.95. The sandwich boxes had sold out when we got there. Baby changing is in a separate room near the toilets by the restaurant.

We had brought a picnic and you're not allowed to eat this in the café, but there are tables outside and you can eat in the aquatheatre.

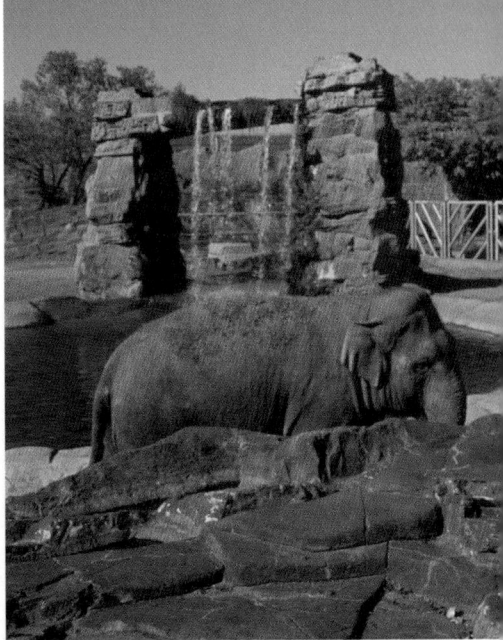

Although Chester Zoo is an expensive day out, it is exactly that 'a day out', there is so much to see you could easily come back for a second or even third visit and still have things to do.

Outside is Octopus Island, a good play area and where you'll also find the otters.

I don't think we missed much and including our lunch we were there for around three hours. You can go round the aquarium as many times as you like, but I didn't feel it's really a full day out.

In my opinion round every corner in Blue Planet there was something to spend money on, whether it's face painting, helium Nemo balloons, photographs, sweets, vending machines or the enormous gift shop – all a nightmare for parents still reeling from the entry fee.

Mon-Fri 10am-5pm Weekends 10am-6pm
Adult £14.50, Child £10.50, Family £48, Groovy Grandparent Ticket £44, Child under 95cm free.
Free car park.
Blue Planet, Kinsey Road, Cheshire CH65 9LF
Tel: 0151 357 8804 www.blueplanetaquarium.com

Bowland Wild Boar Park

This is a great working farm and education centre. You can hand feed deer, llamas and goats and in springtime lambs and chicks can be stroked.

The play area is excellent with a sandpit and diggers, a brilliant zip wire suitable from three years old, which Sebastian loved and a pedal tractor area that is free. There are barrel rides running all year that cost £1, and for the more sedate amongst

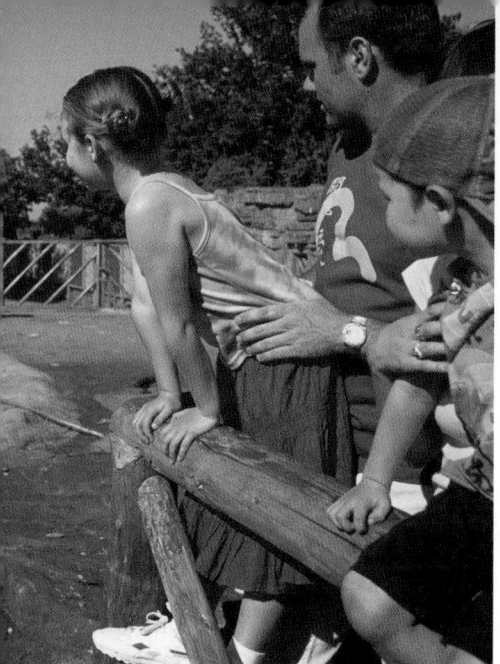

Animals, nature and wildlife

Chester Zoo

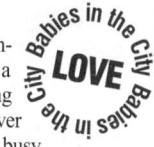

An easy drive to Chester from Manchester and lots of parking made a good start to the day. We were visiting mid-week, during term time and over winter so thankfully it wasn't too busy.

There is so much to see over such a vast area, that you could easily come back for a second visit. In the summer months it does get very busy and unlike the unlimited viewing of the orang-utans that we had, it can be a slow moving walk past with no opportunity to stop and admire.

We had taken a packed lunch and happened to stumble on the Arara Picnic Lodge by the jaguar enclosure just as it started raining. Although not heated it did keep us warm and dry. Children's meals are available at all the restaurants, staff are happy to heat up bottles and there is a microwave available at Café Tsavo near the main entrance.

Highlights of our visit included the orang-utans – they really appeared to try and communicate with us. The jaguars were gorgeous too – in the middle of the Jaguar House there is a branch, which I thought was to add ambience; it took a three year old to point out that in fact leafcutter ants were busy working away carrying leaves – absolutely hypnotic.

My children did get excited at one particular sighting... pointing excitedly as a big yellow JCB digger dug a hole. Honestly I felt like shoving them all in the car there and then!

I really liked the Twilight Zone; I couldn't get Oliver's mum to come in with me as she was terrified, so I went in with all the kids. It is a bit surreal – a big open enclosure with bats flying around. You can feel the movement of the air as they brush past your ear. There were overhanging rocks to walk under and by the end of it even I was spooked, which the children found hilarious! Also well planned was the monkey area. With no cages, it is all set on an island with a small moat and you feel you could just hop over.

The children's play area, Fun Ark, is good for a bit of time out for parents so you can grab a cup of tea while they cavort. There is also face painting available for £4 and a pottery painting studio.

The zoo is a massive 110 acres, a big area to cover and often a long walk between enclosures so I would recommend taking your pushchair with you. Everywhere is accessible and if you forget yours you can hire one from Zoo Mobility at the main entrance for £5 plus a £10 refundable deposit. You can pre-book a pushchair by calling 01244 389482.

Separate baby changing facilities are available at all toilets, which tend to be near the café areas and

us there is a tractor and trailer ride going up through the woodland also for £1. You can then get off and walk through the woods back to the farm or hop back on the tractor.

Being situated in the heart of the Trough of Bowland on the River Hodder there are some great riverside walks which are ideal for children, pushchairs and grandparents. They vary in length from 550-1200 metres. Make sure you don't forget the wellies as it can get very muddy. You are welcome to take a picnic and ramble through Ribble Valley Park alongside the wild boar, longhorn cows and deer, but you may not feed the animals. If you haven't brought your own food then the café serves home cooked dishes and children's meals, with the speciality being home reared wild boar meat sausages and burgers.

Lastly take a look in the eco lodge to see how much electricity is being produced. There is no mains electricity to Bowland, so approximately a third is generated by the huge wind turbine and two solar panels.

Summer: Daily Easter-31st Oct 10.30am-5pm
Winter: Daily 1st Nov-Easter 11am-4pm
Café is open daily during the summer and Fri-Mon during the winter
Summer: Adult £4.50, Child £4, Family Ticket £15, Under 2s free.
Winter: £3.50 for everyone over 2 years old.
There is an 'Honesty Box' when no-one is in attendance.
Bowland Wild Boar Park, Chipping, Preston PR3 2QT
Tel: 01995 61554 www.wildboarpark.co.uk

Animals, nature and wildlife

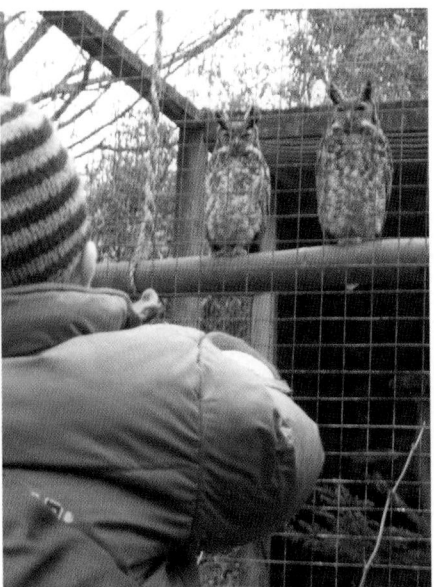

Our two year old has not stopped "twit twooing" since visiting the Chestnut Centre. The conservation park is made up primarily of otters and sixteen types of owls.

The Chestnut Centre Otter, Owl & Wildlife Park

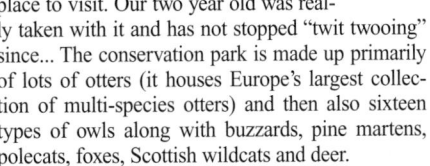

If you fancy a little run out, this delightful park on the Manchester edge of the Peak District is a perfect place to visit. Our two year old was really taken with it and has not stopped "twit twooing" since... The conservation park is made up primarily of lots of otters (it houses Europe's largest collection of multi-species otters) and then also sixteen types of owls along with buzzards, pine martens, polecats, foxes, Scottish wildcats and deer.

A special highlight is Manoki, the UK's only giant otter – he's around 1.5 metres long. Rather brilliantly you get a great view in to his enclosure via a glass wall and he does seem to love performing to a crowd when he's fishing.

Your tour round the park and its animals (which took us about two and a half hours) is via a very picturesque woodland trail dotted with information boards about what you're seeing which would be good for older children. The enclosures are well designed in that you get to see the animals pretty close up and the otters were clearly very happy in their environment. They were incredibly playful which was lovely to watch. We actually took a pram round (the centre describes itself as wheelchair access manageable with fit helpers only) and that was fine because there were two of us to negotiate some awkward areas where there were steps. Be warned, the final leg of the trail back up to the car park is a relatively steep walk through a path in a field!

The centre also contains a café and a gift shop. The café sells simple but delicious food – jacket potatoes, sandwiches or soup. Children's lunch boxes were £2.25, which we thought was good value. High chairs available. Baby changing facilities in the ladies toilets and the café will provide hot water for heating up bottles.

Daily in Autumn and Winter (weekends only in January) 10.30am-Dusk.
Daily in Spring and Summer 10.30am-5.30pm.
Adult £6.50, Child £4.50, Under 2s free.
Family Ticket £20
Chestnut Centre, Chapel-en-le-Frith, High Peak, Derbyshire SK23 0QS
Tel: 01298 814099   www.chestnutcentre.co.uk

Farmer Ted's Farm Park

The joy of Farmer Ted's is that unlike a lot of outdoor farm and theme parks, it's open all year round and there's a fair amount indoors so inclement weather doesn't hold you back.

There's an outdoor adventure playground zoned for the over and under 3s, a pedal tractor park, an excellent indoor sand pit, tractor barrel rides (£1

the main entrance. You can buy nappies from guest services or from vending machines within the toilet.

Lastly to get the children out of the zoo we promised them a trip on the Zoofari monorail; it costs £2 for adults and £1.50 for over 3s and you buy tickets at the machine. If you go from Jubilee Station at the furthest end of the zoo, you whiz back to the entrance and the kids get a last look at the animals, you can't however do a round trip as you must split your journey. It is no problem taking your pushchair on.

A waterbus runs from Easter until autumn though only at weekends during term time. It's a 15 minute trip allowing close up views of some of the animal enclosures; it's the same price as the monorail. You can't take pushchairs on but there is a place to store them.

New for 2009 is a Butterfly house – over 500 butterflies will be housed at a new tropical exhibit, another good indoors escape from dodgy weather.

Winter 10am-4pm, Summer 10am-5pm, Summer holidays 10am-6pm Last admission is one hour before closing. Check website for details. Free parking Peak 4th Apr-1st Nov 2009 Prices unavailable as we were went to press.
Off-peak 3rd Nov 2008-3rd Apr 2009 Adult £11.95, Child £8.95, Family £38, Under 3s £1
Chester Zoo, Cedar House, Caughall Road, Upton-by-Chester, Chester CH2 1LH
Tel: 01244 380 280 www.chesterzoo.org

OUT AND ABOUT

extra and it's weather dependent), a go-kart circuit and a large animal barn with cows, pigs, llamas and ponies amongst others. The farm allows the children to see and take part in demonstrations ranging from milking cows and handling guinea-pigs to grooming the ponies – the children loved taking part.

A highlight is always the tractor ride. Rides leave at various times of the day and involve a tractor pulling an open sided, covered trailer full of straw bales that parents and children sit on. The tour runs around the farm's fields and a talk is given about the animals you see along the way plus there's a bit of a sing-song.

The indoor adventure area is another good feature – it's not enormous but allows another chance for the children to exhaust themselves clambering all over it. There's a separate soft play section as well for the Under 4s. Next door to this is the restaurant – Farmer Ted's Grill (open: 10am-5pm) so you can eat and watch your children play if you wish. It's got a comprehensive children's menu serving sausage in a bun, bread-crumbed chicken and chips and pasta dishes etc for £2.95. There are high chairs and a microwave for heating up baby food. Outside you'll find plenty of picnic tables if you want to bring your own lunch. Toilets are located next to the restaurant with baby changing in the womens' and disabled.

Daily 10am-6pm (closed Tuesdays during term time)
Mon-Fri Adult £2.50, Over 3s £4.50, Under 3s £3.50, Under 1s free
Weekends, School Holidays and June-Sept Adult £4.50, Over 3s £6.50, Under 3s £4, Under 1s free Family Ticket £20.50
Farmer Ted's Farm Park, Flatman's Lane, Downholland, Ormskirk L39 7HW
Tel: 0151 526 0002 www.farmerteds.com

Heaton Park Farm

See Heaton Park on page 18.

Knowsley Safari Park

We visited Knowsley during the Easter holidays, taking our little boys' three year old cousin with us. The safari park driving route snakes for five miles through various open animal enclosures. If it's a quiet day, you can do this at your own pace, and spend time observing the animals. On our trip, we actually drove round the route twice at my children's insistence who were having a whale of a time. I understand from a friend who went on a Bank Holiday however that her tour of the park was one long traffic jam in the heat and her brood got very restless. It is probably best to choose your day to visit carefully if you have young children who may need a toilet break or require food heating. Once you are in your car and on the route,

you can't get out, and whilst throwing yourself to the lions may seem like a preference to sitting in a hot car with screaming children, it isn't an option.

As anyone who has ever been to a safari park will testify, the best part is the monkey enclosure. The monkeys can be avoided if you are the car polishing type, but this definitely precludes us, so we headed in. The animals' antics sent my children and their cousin into a mixture of laughter and tears. A large baboon's bottom in your car window can be funny but a monkey's head suddenly popping into view an inch from your face can be a bit scary for a two year old.

Once out of the car there are still more animals to see on foot including otters and elephants which can be viewed at reasonably close proximity. There are sea-lions who at regular times throughout the day put on a show of diving through hoops. The children loved the theatre of the show, which was well delivered. There is also a small but well stocked farm with all the usual suspects plus a few llamas and bug house, so all in all animal wise Knowsley have it pretty well covered.

We then headed on to the amusement park which we found appropriate for Under 5s. The rides are not included in the entrance price and instead

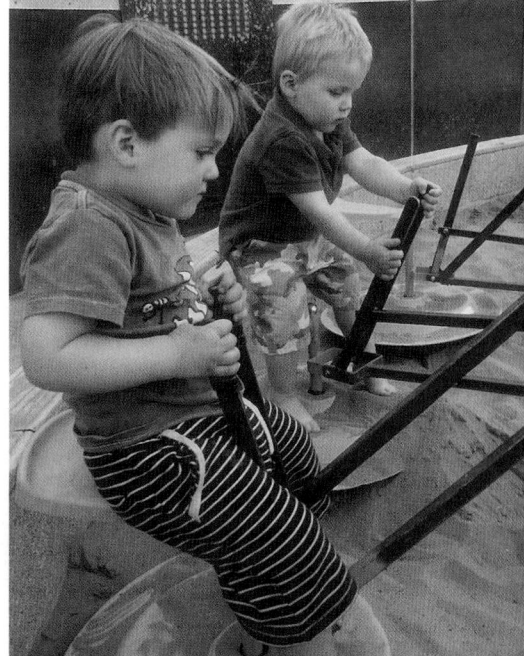

The joy of Farmer Ted's is that it is open all year round. There's an outdoor adventure playground, a pedal tractor park, an excellent indoor sand pit and lots of animals.

Animals, nature and wildlife

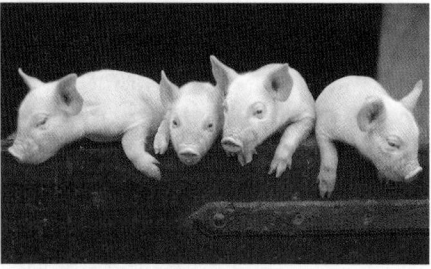

Home Farm at Tatton Park

With a neo-classical mansion and acres of stunning landscaped parkland as its backdrop, this pretty farm probably wins the award for best setting! There's a car park within Tatton Park grounds (charge for car entry to Tatton £4.50) and from here, the farm's about a five minute walk. During most weekends and school holidays there's a Land Train running between the two which is fun to take (small charge) though the amble past the cows and sheep in the fields is just as nice.

At the working farm children can feed the goats and hens; meet the pigs, cows, horses and donkeys and take a peek inside a 1930's cottage. It's not huge but very sweet and our little boy spent the majority of the time transfixed by the rowdy goats who just loved the attention and food they were getting from us. Food is available to buy in the shop (30p for a bag of corn). Another highlight was seeing the adorable baby piglets – children can get a great view of the pigs and piglets through the new glass viewing panels. Home Farm has an impressive pig herd comprising of six rare breeds and as they farrow twice a year it is possible to see a newborn litter each month. Do be aware that much of the farm is cobbled with uneven stones but we were absolutely fine with our pram.

The farm has toilets and there are baby changing facilities. A tuck shop serving ice cream and refreshments is open during high season. The nearest restaurant is back near the car park.

Events do run through the year so keep an eye on the website. One to look out for is lambing weekend at the farm, April 18th-24th 2009.

Low Season: Oct-March, Weekends 11am-4pm (last entry 3pm); High Season, March-Oct, Tues-Sun 12-5pm (last entry 4pm).
Low Season, Adult £4, Under 16s £2, Under 4s free. Family Ticket £10; High Season, Adult £4.50, Under 16s £2.50, Under 4s free. Family ticket £11.50 Totally Tatton Family ticket £17.50 allows entry to the mansion, garden and farm. Can use this ticket on another day if one or more of those attractions aren't visited (car entry must be paid again)
Tatton Park, Knutsford, Cheshire WA16 6QN
Tel: 01625 374435 www.tattonpark.org.uk

books of tickets are purchased from booths dotted around it. Particularly enjoyable was the little train that took us on a lengthy circular tour and allowed views of some of the animals. Amongst other rides there is a bouncy castle, rattlesnake roller coaster, busy bee ride and ranger cars. There are some age and height restrictions.

The restaurant serves a variety of food and drinks at reasonable prices, however we took a picnic and ate it at one of the tables by the otter enclosure.

The admission to Knowsley Safari Park isn't cheap and when you add on the cost of the amusement rides and ice creams it does mount up. However there is a good mixture of things to do here so I would consider it reasonable value for money. It's a nice treat.

Baby Change Facilities are available.

Open all year round. If the weather is very icy or snowy it is closed for safety reasons. The amusement park is closed in Winter for maintenance.
Summer: 1st Mar-31st Oct 10am
Last entry to Safari Drive 4pm
Winter: 1st Nov-28th Feb 10.30am
Last entry to Safari Drive 3pm
Adult £12, Child £9, Family ticket £37, Pedestrians £7 per person (but you might get eaten!), Under 3s free.
Amusement Rides: £1.50 per ticket, £1 per ticket for 50 or more (but you would have to be insane!!!!!!)
Wristbands for amusement park £9
Knowsley Safari Park, Prescot, Merseyside L34 4AN
Tel: 0151 430 9009 www.knowsley.com

Reddish Vale Farm

From the outside Reddish Vale Farm looks quite small, no impressive tractor rides or bales of hay, but this is why I liked it. For the nought to five age group this is the perfect farm, it is not huge and therefore felt very safe. Nobody could wander off and get lost. There were plenty of famyard animals, ducks, pigs, horses, sheep, donkeys and goats plus a lovely petting area with guinea pigs and rabbits. All the animals were easy to see and they had even made low windows in the pigsty. Buckets of carrots to feed the animals are 50p.

For a final workout there was a bouncy castle and a bouncy slide also 50p for five minutes though in quiet times you can go on for as long as you like. Plus there is a selection of ride on tractors and trailers that were free. On Sunday's from 1-3pm there are pony rides for £1.50.

The tearooms are open every weekend throughout the year. Children's meals are available from £2.50 for either a burger, chicken nuggets or hot dog and chips. A bottle warmer and high chairs are available. Baby changing is in the disabled toilet

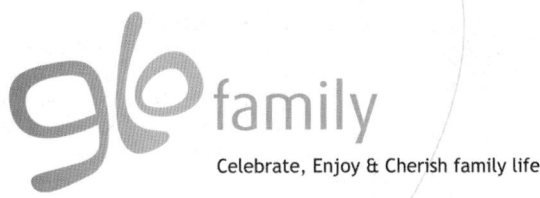
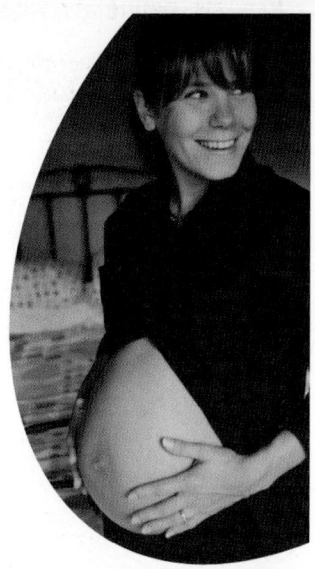
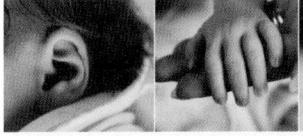 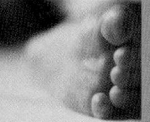
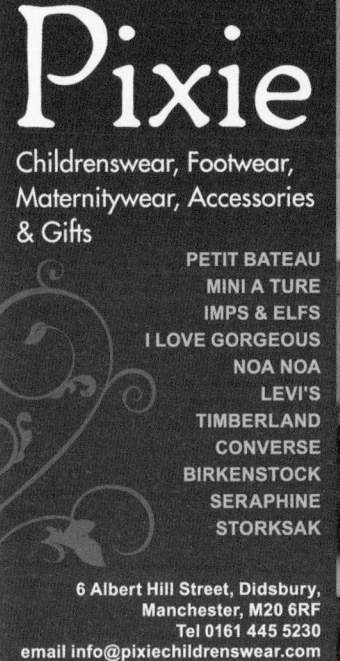
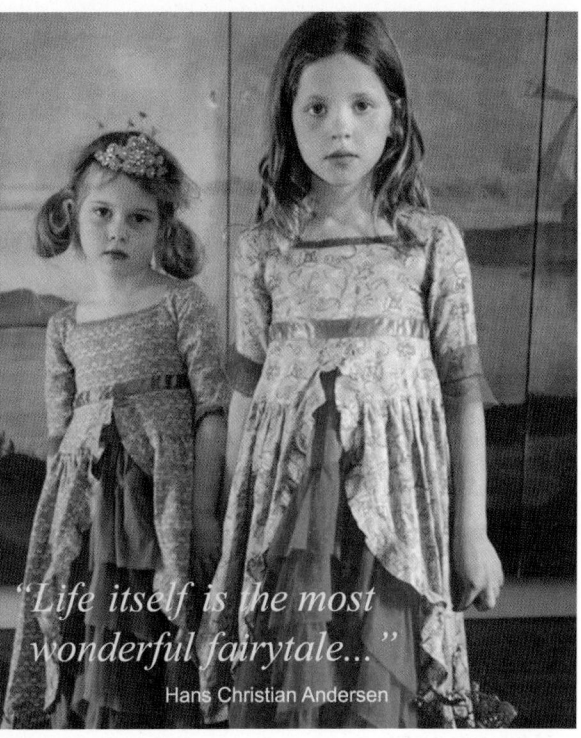

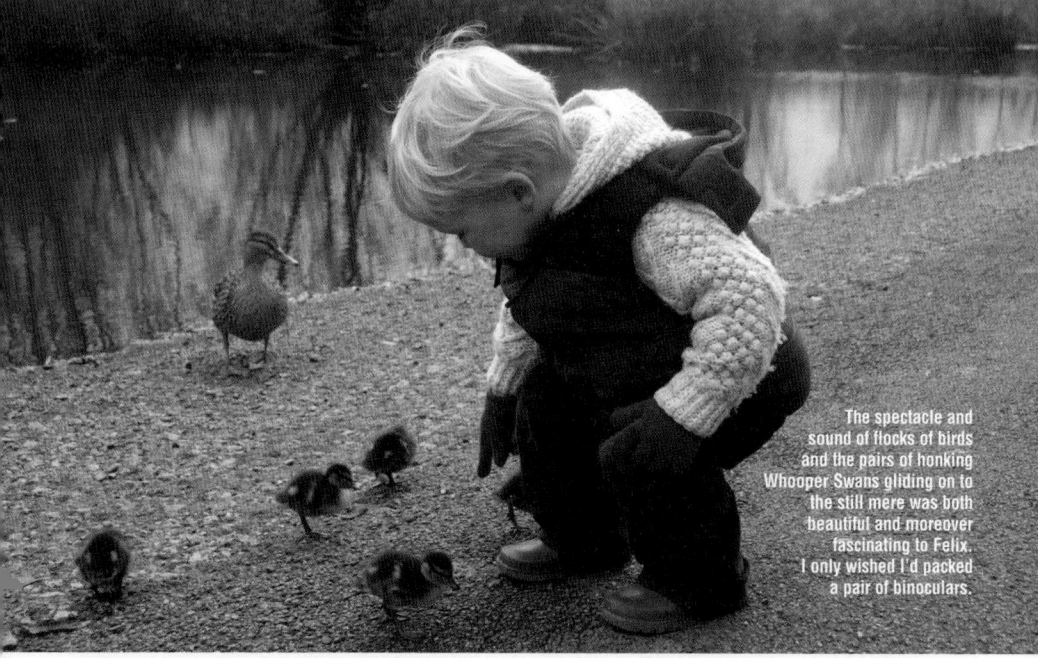

The spectacle and sound of flocks of birds and the pairs of honking Whooper Swans gliding on to the still mere was both beautiful and moreover fascinating to Felix. I only wished I'd packed a pair of binoculars.

Martin Mere Wetland Centre

Babies in the City LOVE

Martin Mere is a wildfowl and wetlands reserve allowing visitors' access to animals in a natural and tranquil environment.

I went with my 22 month old son, Felix, in November and later learnt that this is one of the more exciting times of year in the bird watching calendar as it is when migratory birds depart and arrive for winter.

We rolled up mid morning by car after a journey taking approximately 1hr 10 mins from south Manchester. The distance between the M61 exit and the centre was a little longer than I had anticipated but it was a scenic drive, and very well signposted. Entry was via a visitor centre which also houses a restaurant, gift shop and toilets. We had a quick tea and juice stop in the restaurant, where we bought a bag of crusty bread duck food for 50p, before exploring the wetlands.

The wetlands is initially set out in a series of fenced areas, linked by a circular paved route, with birds from different continents of the world. My son toddled between the continents poking his crusty bread at the birds and was particularly taken by the Magpie Geese from Australasia which tickled his fingers, and also the stepping stones across the pond of the Oriental section. Also in this part of the centre is the beaver hide. Unfortunately we didn't see any beavers on this visit – this may have been because my son scared them off shouting "beefers" at the top of his voice.

A pre-recorded web cam of the beavers can be watched in the hide however to avoid too much disappointment.

On the periphery is the mere and the reed beds which are overlooked by a series of hides, the most impressive of which is the Harrier Hide. This is built in wood to look like a Harrier jet, with an interesting history of the wetlands on the pathway, and floor to ceiling windows inside which my son liked. The spectacle and sound of flocks of birds and the pairs of honking Whooper Swans gliding on to the still mere were both beautiful and moreover fascinating to my little boy. He was quite content sat on a stool watching and pointing for well over 30 minutes. I only wished I'd packed a pair of binoculars.

We ate lunch at the restaurant, where hot food is served from 11.45am-2.30pm. I settled for a bacon butty which was delicious and Felix had a child's lunch box, which consisted of a sandwich, fruit, a juice and some crisps for £3.50. A hot children's meal was available for the same price. We ended the visit in the play area, which after an enjoyable day was an added bonus. It's accessed via a tunnel and divided into two parts dependant on age, both with a good range of equipment. Surrounding the playground were plenty of benches where you could comfortably sit and watch.

In the spring a hatchery/nursery is open and baby chicks can be viewed up close, which we'll definitely go back to see!

Unisex baby change facilities available. High chairs in the restaurant and staff were happy to heat baby food and milk.

Daily Nov-Feb 9.30am-5pm (last admission 4pm)
March-Oct 9.30am-5.30am (last admission 5pm)
Adult £8.75, Child £4.30, Under 4s free. Family tickets £23.50.
Car parking free
WWT Martin Mere Wetland Centre, Fish Lane, Burscough, Lancashire L40 0TA
Tel: 01704 895181 www.wwt.org.uk

by the entrance to the farm. See page 21 for information on Reddish Vale Country Park.

28th Feb-24th Oct and 5th Dec-24th Dec, Weekends 11am-4pm; School Holidays and Bank Holidays Daily 11am-4pm (Stockport holidays can differ from Manchester so check first)
Adult £2.50, Child £1.50, Under 3s free. Cash only.
Tearooms: Sat 9am-4pm, Sun 9.30am-4pm. Open daily in school holidays 9.30am-4pm.
Tel: 0161 480 1645
Reddish Vale Farm, Reddish Vale Road, Reddish,
Stockport SK5 7HE
Tel: 0161 480 1645
www.reddishvalefarm.co.uk

SEA LIFE

Well worth a visit is the Sea Life centre on Blackpool's Golden Mile. We went out of season and during term time, which made for a lovely relaxing trip with no fighting for a glimpse of the fishies. It's not massive and will take about an hour for a pleasant mooch round.

First up is the touch pool – an open rock pool filled with various sea creatures that the staff help you handle. We thought the staff here were excellent. A young woman completely engaged with our boys as she helped them hold a starfish, giving them lots of bite-size nuggets of information along the way. From there it's on to the aquarium itself. The fifty-odd tanks are all at a good height for little ones, so there's no straining to see the array of fish within. Our boys were counting sharks, rays, seahorses and piranhas within minutes.

A big favourite was the ray pool. The boys had fun walking over the pool on the walkway that criss-crossed above it, which gives you a great view of the fish being fed by staff. In fact, the only bit not to meet with full approval was the talking pirate hologram by the aquatheatre. This was deemed "a bit scary".

Inevitably the summer months are busy, but don't be deterred. The Sea Life centre puts on free additional attractions, like face painting, badge making etc to ensure the wait is never boring. The café is quite small and has no outside space. It does however, have a mini soft play area and ball pit, which kept our lot happy for a good half hour. When the café is quiet, you're welcome to eat your

packed lunch there. Menu included jacket potatoes at £2.25 and hot dogs at £1.95. A meal deal including sandwich, crisps and drink cost £3.95. There are high chairs and the café will readily heat up bottles. The only toilets are near the ray pool and baby-changing facilities are found in the disabled cubicle.

If you have a pram, you'll need to walk back to the beginning of the tour to use the lift. Otherwise, you'll be faced with a huge flight of stairs at the end.

A criticism we'd heard related to the high cost of admission. However Sea Life frequently offer excellent promotional discounts so it's worth scouring the internet and contacting the tourist office before you go. Plus see our fantastic offer on p95 of £5 off entry pice per person!

Nearest parking is on Bonny Street, directly behind the centre.
Daily 10am-3pm or 4pm dependent on time of year.
Adult £12.50, Child 3-14 years £9.95, Under 3s free
SEA LIFE, Blackpool Promenade, Blackpool, Lancashire FY1 5AA
Tel: 01253 621258
www.sealifeeurope.com

TOP FIVE ANIMAL ATTRACTIONS

Stockley Farm
Attractions galore from tractor rides to bottle feeding baby animals. A highlight for any child.

Chester Zoo
One of the UK's top zoos with over 7000 animals and 400 species, it's a great day out for the whole family.

Chestnut Centre
A unique wildlife park which contains one of Europe's largest groups of otters and owls. Well worth a visit.

Reddish Vale
A variety of farmyard animals to look at and touch. Ideal for toddlers.

Martin Mere
Home to rare and endangered swans, flamingoes and beavers. A first class, year-round, wetland wildife attraction.

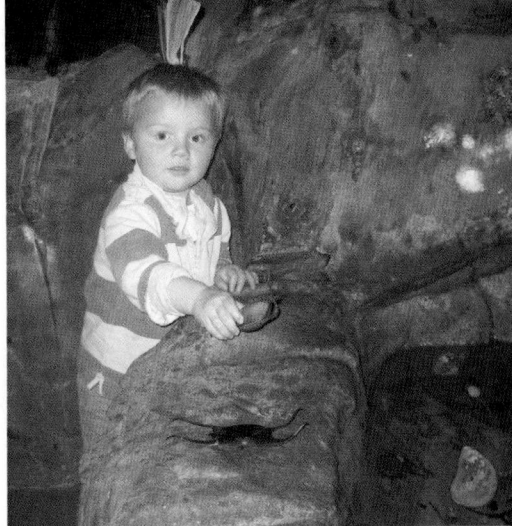

The touch pool at Sea Life – an open rock pool filled with various sea creatures that the staff help you handle.

Animals, nature and wildlife

Smithills Open Farm

The main attraction at Smithills Farm is the big barn – inside the noise is incredible and the smell is pretty overwhelming too! You can buy bags of animal feed for 50p, which is a must as literally every type of farm animal is available for you to stroke, feed and pet. We saw cows, calves, pigs, sheep, chickens, plus some overzealous goats that managed to grab the food bag off Will and eat the whole lot!

Thankfully in the same barn and perfect for a quick distraction there's a seated pets corner, probably our children's favourite bit. They loved holding baby rabbits, guinea pigs and even tiny chicks – I was trying to look calm, fully expecting a child to drop one or accidentally squeeze the poor thing a bit hard, but staff are on hand to help with the squirming animals.

Baby changing is in the disabled toilet, which could do with a bit of an upgrade.

Every day at 1pm you can watch the cows being milked in the main barn although it does get a bit smelly! During the summer and at weekends you can help feed the lambs.

Lastly there is a small vivarium, which if you don't like snakes you can easily avoid. The snakes are only brought out for demonstrations but if you really want to hold one you can ask a member of staff and they are happy to oblige.

Mon-Sun 10am-5pm
Adult £5, Child over 2 £4, Under 2s free
Smithills Open Farm, Smithills Dean Road, Bolton, Lancashire BL1 7NS
Tel: 01204 595765 www.smithillsopenfarm.co.uk
Bus to: 501 (Captains Clough Road), 519 (Lightbounds Road).
Train to: Bolton, then bus.

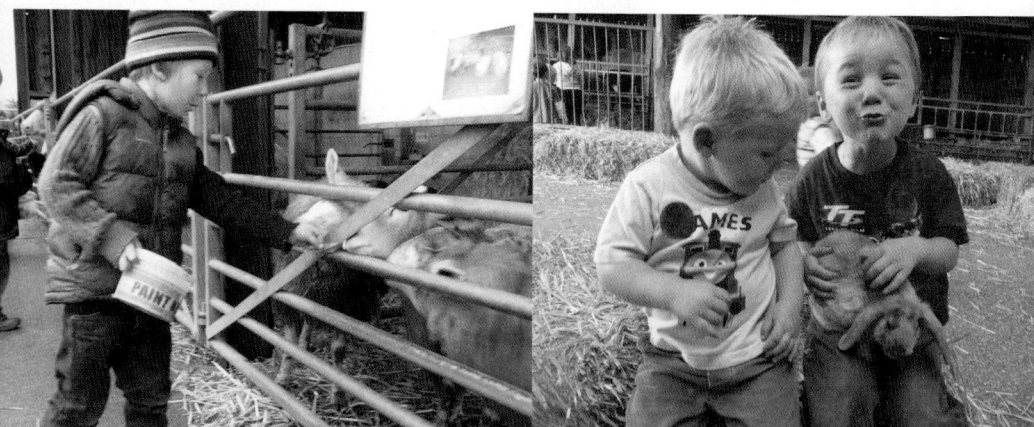

Left page: Ollie feeding the animals carrots at Reddish Vale Farm, it is small and feels very safe. The seated pets corner was probably Harry and Sam's favourite bit at Smithills Farm. They loved holding baby rabbits, guinea pigs and even tiny chicks. Right page: Sasha got to feed the goats enormous bottles of milk at Stockley Farm.

Outside and up in the top fields there are plenty of animals still to see and friendly pigs trot along after you as you visit llamas, alpacas and deer. There is a large adventure playground for older children, an old tractor to climb on plus some ride-on tractors. A smaller play area for toddlers is by the main entrance. Donkey rides are available every day for £1 a go. Plus in the summer and weekends during winter, tractor-trailer rides are £1 per person. There are two bouncy castles inside which are free with no time restrictions.

There is a good size café with highchairs and children's meals are £2 for chicken nuggets/fish fingers/sausages with chips. They are happy to warm up milk or baby food. You are welcome to bring a picnic – there are plenty of tables outside, and if it is raining there are some indoors.

Stockley Farm

A visit to Stockley Farm starts from the moment you park your car. A tractor and trailer are waiting in the car park to transport you the short journey down to the farm. Taking a pushchair on wasn't a problem; the drivers are happy to help you and your little ones clamber up to sit on bales of hay.

When you arrive you're not exactly sure what to do first, but what does strike you is how well kept the farm is. First off we hit the sheds to see the cows and calves, pigs, goats and lambs. We then moved on to the pets corner, where my boys enjoyed stroking baby rabbits, guinea pigs and chicks – I was amazed at how gentle they were.

There is a brilliant sand pit with at least half a dozen mechanical diggers and loads of toys.

Babies in the City LOVE

There's also an old tractor, a climbing frame and slide. In the large barn there is another sand pit with a cement mixer, a small soft play area, ride on pedal tractors, a bouncy castle and the boys' favourite – enormous bales of hay to roll around in.

Throughout the day there are opportunities to feed the animals. This is very popular and does get busy. While you sit on hay bales, skittish goats are brought in for the children to feed; they work slowly down the barn with enormous bottles of milk so everyone gets a turn. In the summer, sheep races are held plus at weekends, bird of prey displays.

For lunch there is a spacious café with loads of highchairs offering home made cakes and sandwich boxes for children. There is a microwave and bottle warmer for baby food and bottles. We'd brought a picnic and you'll find plenty of tables either outside in the play area or inside the barn.

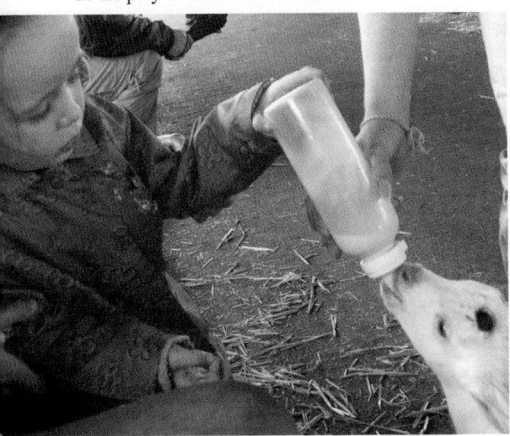

The disabled toilet has a pull down changing table and a nappy dispensing machine. There is also a heated mother and baby room with a comfy chair for breastfeeding and a changing mat.

At 3.30pm every day you can watch the cows being milked via a special purpose-built viewing gallery. When it was time to leave, the only way to get mine out was the promise of another tractor ride back to the car.

Weekends 22nd Mar-25th Oct 11am-5pm; every Weds from 25th March-15th July 1-5pm; daily in school holidays 11am-5pm, 28th Nov-20th Dec 11am-5pm
Adult £7, Child £6, Under 2s free, Family ticket £25
Joint Tickets for Stockley Farm and Arley Hall and Gardens are also available.
Stockley Working Farm, Stockley Farm, Arley, Northwich, Cheshire CW9 6LZ
Tel: 01565 777323 www.stockleyfarm.co.uk

Wythenshawe Farm
See Wythenshawe Park on page 22.

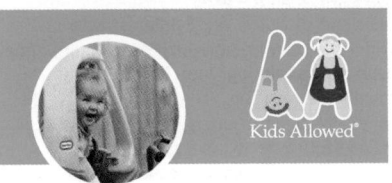
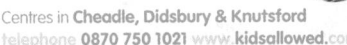
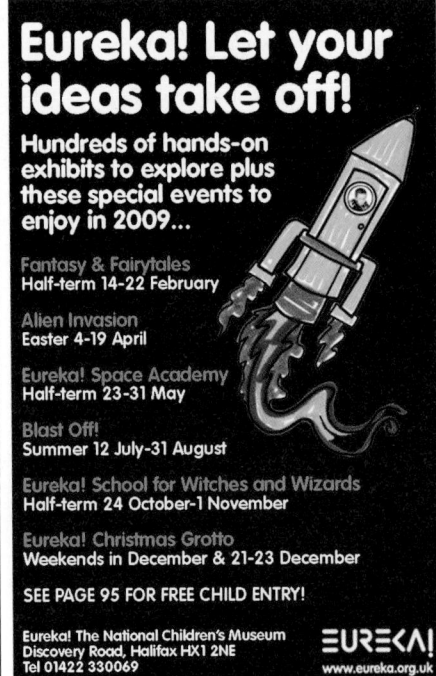

Step back in time and lose yourself in the splendour of North West past. Gorgeous grounds, romantic houses and splendid deer parks – a stunning escape from city life.

Country estates

Arley Hall and Gardens

This is a great place to go with young children if you are a garden lover. We have visited both in summer and at Christmas and have found Arley a treasure trove for young and old alike. With the car parked it's a short stroll along an impressive tree-lined avenue. On entering the estate via the gift shop, you'll find a cobbled stable yard bordered by the restaurant and toilet facilities. In the warmer months several tables are set out for eating here. The cobbles are a bit awkward with a pram but the rest of Arley is very accessible. Passing under the clock tower, which houses a bell that to the delight of the children is rung regularly, you are greeted with the splendid hall. The hall itself, whilst beautiful, is probably a bit dull for little ones; but it isn't large and sprawling so a tour round can be short if you wish. At Christmas the hall comes to life with floral displays and activities for children. My three-year-old son made a beautiful floral table display last year that we proudly used on Christmas Day, and we all learnt about Victorian Christmas food in the kitchens.

The gardens are magnificent. Clearly a lot of love and care has gone into their design and maintenance. For under fives they are as much fun as you want to make them. Separated into 'rooms' of colour or design there are plenty of pathways and hidey-holes for playing chase or hide and seek. Situated in the gardens and surrounded by shrub roses is a little half-timbered cottage, built in the mid 19th century, as a place for the family living at Arley at the time to enjoy afternoon tea. Today it is open to go inside, and with its tiny proportions makes it a perfect place to play house.

The children also love watching the fish in the fish garden and try their best to get wet in the several fountains dotted about. There are plenty of open spaces where they can run and jump, and with the grass being manicured and dog poop free it makes a perfect place to roll around or kick a ball. If you are looking for something a bit more rugged, there is a woodland walk on the other side of the hall, which we found manageable with slow walkers and prams.

For refreshments there is the restaurant housed in The Tudor Barn. It's a terrific building and between 12 and 3pm serves a good selection of food. The kids menu includes cheese sandwiches for £3 or pizza for £3.95. There weren't many high chairs when we went but apparently plans are afoot to change this. The staff will happily heat up baby jars and bottles. Alternatively, if you want to take your own food there is a pleasant picnic area situated round a new and well-designed playhouse. This doubles as a climbing frame and incorporates among other things noughts and crosses, and a long rope to thread in and out of many different holes. It certainly captured my children's imagination. We'll definitely be going back to Arley and this year hope to make it to the annual horse trials in May or the outdoor theatre performance in August. Baby changing available.

Gardens, chapel, grounds and plant nursery open Tues-Sun and Bank Holidays 20th Mar-27th Sep, Sat and Sun Oct 11am-5pm (last entry 4.30pm). Hall open Tues, Sun and Bank Holidays 22nd March-27th Sep, Sun Oct 12noon-5pm (last entry 4.30pm). Garden performance of Charlotte's Web 23rd Aug 2009. Parking free. Adult £5.50 for Gardens, £2.50 for Hall; Under 16s £2 for Gardens, £1 for Hall; Under 5s free, Family Ticket £13 for Gardens, £7 for Hall. Tickets can be bought in conjunction with Stockley Farm (see page 38). Arley Hall & Gardens, Northwich, Cheshire CW9 6NA Tel: 01565 777353 www.arleyhallandgardens.com

Bramall Hall Park

Just outside Bramhall village near Cheadle Hulme, Bramall Hall Park is 70 acres of breathtaking parkland surrounding one of Cheshire's grandest black and white timber-framed buildings. There is a pay and display car park, 70p for one hour, £1 for two hours, but entrance to the parkland is free.

Designed in the style of Capability Brown, the park offers magnificent vistas from the Hall, which is perched on the brow of a hill.

Grass terraces lead downhill to three substantial man-made ponds and the diverted River Ladybrook, which snakes its way through the grounds. The ponds contain islands designed to resemble a Himalayan wilderness. I'm not so sure they are that, but they certainly create a stunning landscape. Well-marked, tarmac paths run through the formal gardens near the Hall and the woodlands beyond, so it's pretty pram-friendly. There are three main bridges so crossing between the sides of the river is easy and a leisurely stroll takes less than an hour. The park's full of good climbing trees and the river itself has safe shelving banks so children can play at the water's edge as well as cross to parts of the 'Himalayan islands'. Wellies are definitely strongly recommended!

Back up at the main house there is a large gated

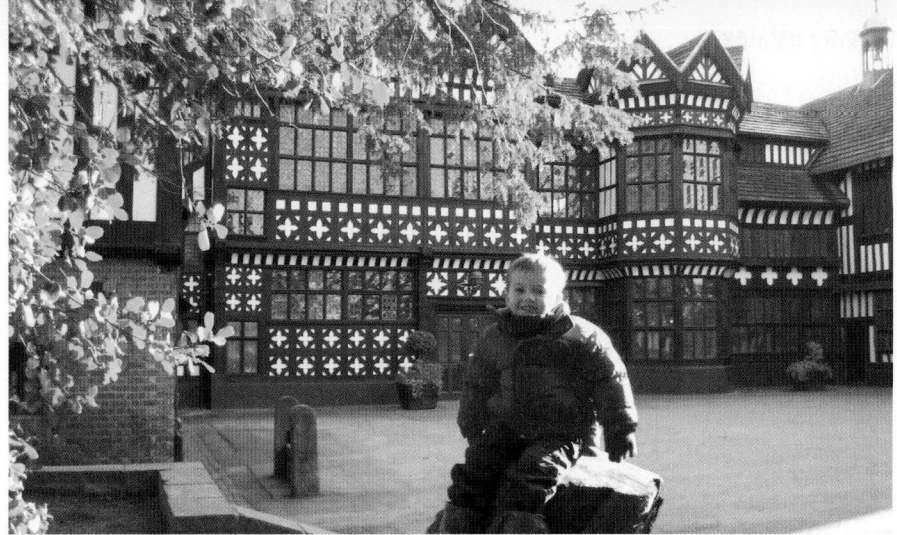

Will at Bramall Hall, one of Cheshire's grandest black and white timber-framed buildings situated within 70 acres of parkland.

children's playground, aimed at the under eights, plus four climbing frames on a grassed area for the older ones. There is also a grassed slope down to the water that is great for 'rolling'! The Hall is open for guided tours only. We didn't go in, but it looked beautiful.

There is a lovely café in the courtyard by the Hall, which has an enclosed outer seating area as well as an indoor section. It offers a reasonably priced selection of hot food and snacks as well as a lunch box for children with a choice of what's included (£2.10 for four items or £2.50 for five).

There are toilets within the park grounds close to the car park, in the café and in the Hall. Baby changing is in the disabled toilets in the café.

Bramall Hall: Sun-Thurs 1st Apr-30th Sep 1-5pm, Fri and Sat 1-4pm, Bank Holidays 11am-4pm; Tues-Sun 1st Oct-1st Jan 1-4pm, Bank Holidays 11am-4pm.
Café: 1st Apr-30th Sep 10am-5.15pm, 1st Oct-31st March 10am-4.15pm
Adult £3.95, Child £2.95, Under 5s free.
Tickets can be bought in conjunction with Staircase House and Stockport Air Raid Shelters (see page 11).
Bramall Hall, Bramhall Park, off Hall Road, Bramhall, Stockport SK7 3NX
Tel: 0161 485 3708 www.bramallhall.org.uk
Bus to: Bramhall Lane South (307, 308, 377, 378).
Train to: Stockport, then bus.

Chatsworth House

Whilst the road from Manchester and particularly North Manchester may be a long and winding route, it is definitely worth making a day trip to Chatsworth. I have been with my boys in both summer and winter and each trip has been a success.

The farmyard and adventure playground are superb. These two features alone make it worth the trip. At the farmyard you can stroke the guinea pigs, watch the cows being milked, sit on a tractor,

and see, among other favourites, the shire horses, piglets and goats. The adventure playground can be accessed by a child-sized tunnel and ladder.

Water and sand are always a winning combination for children and the playground at Chatsworth does it brilliantly. Water can be drawn from a passing stream by turning a large metal corkscrew which then empties into a series of channels, cogs and funnels, before seeping out into troughs dug by children in the sand. On a summer visit my boys spent at least an hour in the sandpit, digging, paddling, splashing, turning and damming. There are also sit-on diggers which scoop out the sand and buckets on chains to hoist it up to a wooden platform. There were buckets and spades available to use on our visits but it may be worth taking a set with you, along with a pair of wellies and a change of clothes.

The rest of the playground is set in the woods and is divided into age appropriate sections with wooden rope bridges, slides, nets and trampolines. There are picnic tables in both the playground and farmyard areas. There is also a modern simple café set over a well-stocked gift shop selling pasties, sandwiches, ice-creams, and drinks etc. The whole area is easily accessible for pushchairs and wheel-chairs. Look out for family activity and seasonal days at the farm.

Chatsworth House is not purely for the children – it caters for the parents as well. Visitors can treat themselves to a luxurious afternoon tea in the stables or a browse around the fabulous gift and garden shops. If that doesn't appeal, then there are beautiful gardens with a cascade fountain to paddle in and of course the magnificent Chatsworth house itself. Alternatively try and coincide your trip with

Country estates

one of the many visiting events such as the
Sculpture Exhibition in the gardens. Now in its
third year, it hosts works from artists as celebrated
as Henry Moore and Damien Hirst. Chatsworth
also lays on seasonal events, for example during the
Christmas holidays there was carol singing, a brass
band and a tour of the festively decorated house.

Food outlets, cafés, toilets and paid parking are
all available, and there are baby changing facilities
throughout the estate.

*Park open all year. House, Gardens and Farmyard
open 11th March-23rd Dec (car park shut during
closed season). Last admission one hour before closing.
House and shops open 11am-5.30pm; Garden open
11am-6pm; Farmyard and adventure playground open
10.30am-5.30pm; Carriage House restaurant and
Stables grill and drinks open 10.15am-5pm. Hot food
served at lunchtime; The Cavendish Rooms open
11am-4.30pm. Hot food served at lunchtime.
Discovery Pass valid for one visit to the House and two
visits to the garden and/or farmyard, all within seven
days: Adult £17.60, Child £11, Family Ticket £52.80.
Farmyard and Adventure Playground:
Adult £5.50, Child £5.80, Family Ticket £21.45 (look
out for discount tickets online).
Chatsworth House, Bakewell, Derbyshire DE45 1PP
Tel: 01246 565300 www.chatsworth.org
Trains run from Manchester and Stockport to Matlock and then
there is a connecting bus service to Chatsworth.*

Dunham Massey

Dunham Massey is a personal favourite for easy,
enjoyable walks. The grounds of this country estate
are beautiful – a stunning mix of parkland and
maintained gardens (you have to pay extra to get
into these unless you're a NT member). There are
plenty of deer roaming free and you can get close
for the children to have a good look. A moat
surrounding the early Georgian house is full of
ducks and swans to feed, whilst nearby rabbits hop
around. I spent a lot of time here when Will was a
baby as there are no steep hills and the wide paths
make it ideal pushchair terrain. Now he is older

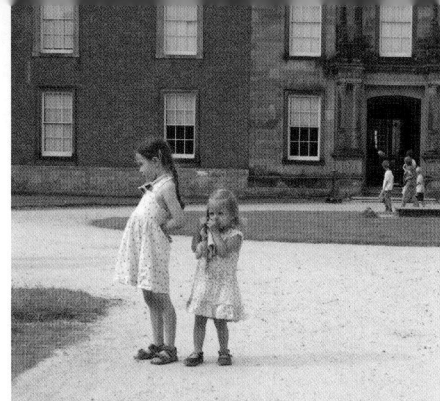

**Sasha and Sofia at Dunham Massey. A moat surrounds the
early Georgian house and deer roam free around the estate.**

there are loads of broken tree trunks lining the walk
which are perfect for climbing over. The other
aspect that is a big hit is the sawmill, where the
giant waterwheel has been restored to full working
order.

There's a designated picnic area outside but if
you haven't packed your own the restaurant in
the converted stables does great home-cooked food,
including an irresistible cake selection. 'Trustyboxes'
containing a ham or cheese roll, a piece of fresh
fruit, a jaffa cake bar and an orange juice are
available for children for £2.95, as well as small
portions of the hot meals on offer (£3.50-£4.50).
They also serve baby deli food for 0-10 months,
pure fruit ice cream lollies and Innocent smoothies.
There's a large separate room just off the main
dining area specifically aimed at families. It has high
chairs and toys, so it doesn't matter as much if the
kids run riot there. Also in this room you'll find a
baby unit with a microwave and bottle warmer.
There's lift access throughout and baby changing is
in the main toilet block adjacent to the restaurant.

The house is worth a look if you've got older
children or easy-going babies. But it's perhaps less
interesting for toddlers and you can't really take
prams inside. However, front-carrying baby slings

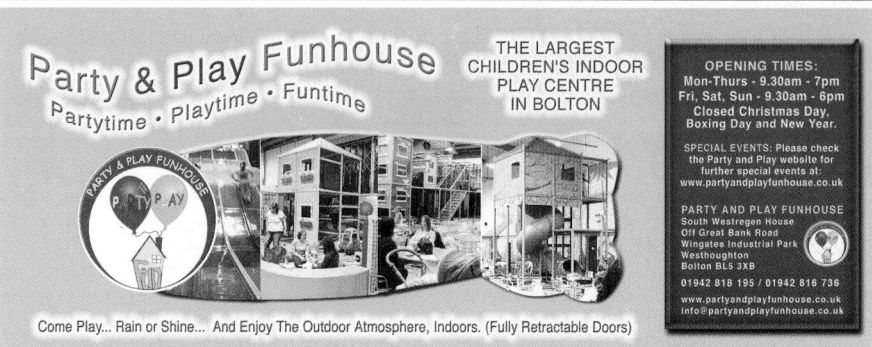

Lyme Park

Lyme Park is a stunning mansion house that resembles an extravagant Italianate palace surrounded by gardens, moorland and ancient deer park. It was used as the setting for the 1995 TV version of Jane Austen's Pride and Prejudice starring Colin Firth. If you go hoping to see Mr Darcy appearing handsomely from the lake, prepare to be disappointed, but if you are looking for somewhere to take the children where they can run around in beautiful surroundings then Lyme Park fits the bill.

It's an ideal venue for meeting friends with children, and is perfect for picnics. After paying the parking entry fee, you proceed down a long scenic driveway with the imposing view of the house ahead, to the car park which is positioned within easy access of everything. There are plenty of picnic areas and lots of open space for the children to explore. Heading towards the timber yard there is a lovely stream and pond, which makes an ideal paddling pool in the warm weather. On the opposite side of the pond, over a bridge, we found a steep bank to scramble up and plenty of fallen trees to climb on. The pretty timber yard housed a coffee shop, toilets and plant shop.

The highlight for the children was the extensive play area. Built from wood with a bark floor, it is nestled in amongst the trees, creating much-needed shade on a hot day. It is really well designed, with three different areas catering for all age groups. A particular favourite with the under fives seems to be a piece of equipment that acts like a set of scales – children sit on a small seat suspended from a rope that is counter-balanced by another seat and rope, creating a unique see-saw effect.

We ended our visit with a short stroll in the deer park but by that stage little legs were getting weary and so we didn't last long, although we did catch a glimpse of one of the fallow deer that roam freely.

The most obvious structure in the park other than the house is a tower called the Cage, which stands on a hill to the east of the approach driveway. I think it looks like a cross between The Tower of London and a castle.

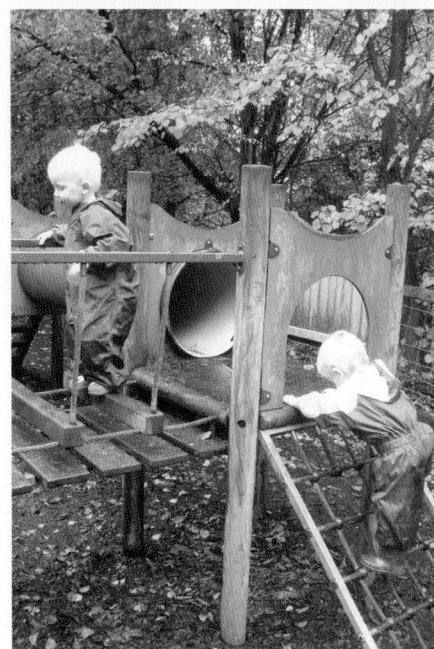

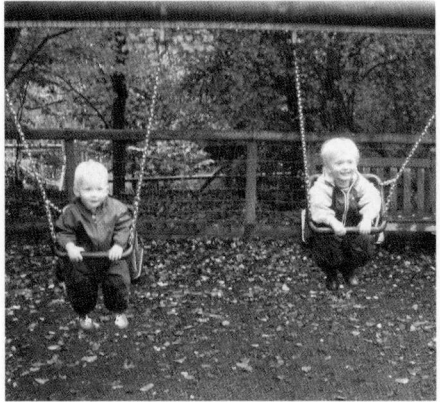

One of the highlights at Lyme Park is the extensive play area. Built from wood with a bark floor, it is really well designed, with three different areas catering for all ages.

It isn't open all the time and the route to it is not pram friendly. It was originally a hunting lodge then later used as a park-keeper's cottage and as a lock-up for prisoners. There isn't much inside except a spiral staircase to climb, but the views towards Manchester are spectacular. There was also a large wooden 3D jigsaw of the Cage for children to play with, which fascinated my four-year-old.

The house itself is also worth a visit – it has a wonderful collection of tapestries, clocks and beautifully furnished rooms. The Victorian garden has roses, sunken parterre and a reflection lake.

Baby change facilities are available.

House/restaurant/shop open: Mon-Sun 14th Mar-31st Oct 11am-5pm (closed Weds/Thurs). House by guided tour only between 11am-12noon. Numbers restricted.
Park open all year from 8am. Garden, as house except open daily 14th Mar-1st Nov, and weekends 7th Nov-20th Dec. Timber Yard Coffee Shop open daily 28th Feb-13th Mar 12-4pm; 14th Mar-1st Nov 10.30am-5pm.
Admission prices at time of going to press only available for 2008. Car entry £4.60 per car. Pedestrians free.
House and Garden: Adult £7.60, Child £3.80, Family £19.
House only: Adult £5.60, Child £2.80.
Garden only: Adult £4.80, Child £2.40.
Lyme Park, Disley, Stockport, Cheshire SK12 2NR
Tel: 01663 762023 www.nationaltrust.org.uk
Bus to: Buxton Road (199). Train to: Disley.

and hip-carrying infant seats are available for loan.

Whilst in the Dunham area you may want to think about paying a visit to Ash Farm, which produces ice cream that must rate as some of the best in the world! The mother and daughter team of Mrs Pennington and Mrs Ogden create flavours as diverse as fruit cake, lavender and ginger, in varying quantities ranging from a simple cone or tub to two litre containers ideal for the freezer. The ice cream shop is open daily 12-5pm (12-6pm in summer and on fine days) and there is a pleasant enclosed garden with tables and chairs in which to sit and gorge!

Ash Farm, Station Road, Dunham Massey WA14 5SG
Tel: 0161 928 1230
Dunham Massey Park open daily summer (28th Feb-1st Nov) 9am-7.30pm; daily winter 9am-5pm.
Stables Restaurant open daily summer 10.30am-5pm (hot food 12-12.30pm); daily winter 10.30am-4pm.
House open summer Sat-Wed 12noon-4.30pm.
Garden re-opens 28th Feb daily 11am-5pm.
House & Garden: Adult £8.50, Child £4.25, Under 5s free, Family ticket £21.25. Garden only: Adult £6, Child £3, Under 5s free. Car Park £4.
Dunham Massey (National Trust Property), Altrincham, Cheshire WA14 4SJ
Tel: 0161 941 1025 www.nationaltrust.org.uk
Bus to: Woodhouse Lane (5 or 38 from Altrincham Interchange).
Tram to: Altrincham, then bus. Train to: Altrincham, then bus.

Quarry Bank Mill and Styal Estate

It was with some trepidation that I ventured to Styal Mill. Memories of sleeping through the Industrial Revolution element of school history lessons coupled with a less than inviting write-up in the National Trust handbook meant I wasn't exactly keen.

The reality far exceeded my expectations. This is a great place to go on a rainy day and if it does turn out nice, the gardens are beautiful and the walk down by the River Bollin is great for pushchairs and toddlers. New for 2009 are children's garden tracker packs, free to borrow from the garden steward in the hut. There is a good play area at the start of the walk plus, as an added incentive, a small café selling ice-lollies, cakes and cups of tea.

Inside the mill, it is pretty impressive. You can't take a pram as you start at the top and wind your way down, but shoulder seats for babies and hip carriers for toddlers are available for a deposit of £5. These can be collected at the Mill entrance. There are interactive exhibits and as you walk around, guides in traditional costume will give you demonstrations and potted histories of certain pieces of equipment. Be warned, if you have a child who doesn't tolerate a lot of noise, this is not the place for you. When the machines are running, the volume is

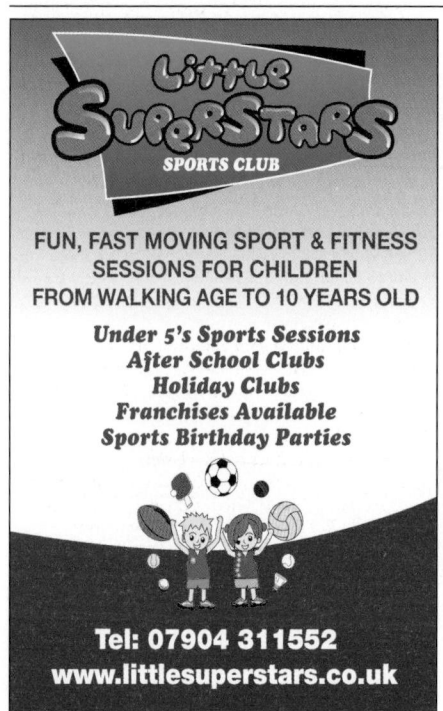

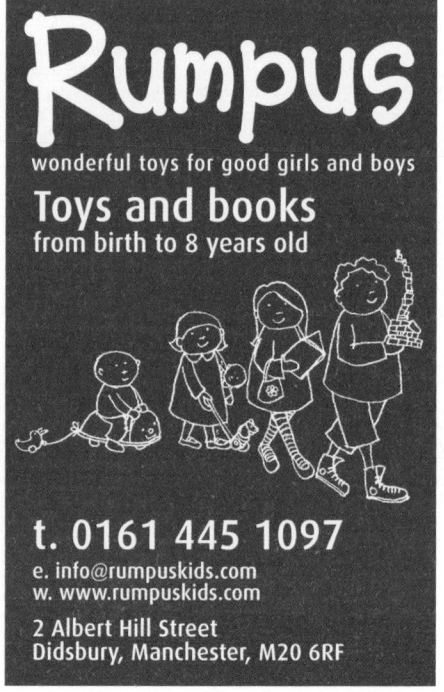

Tatton Park

Tatton Park is one of Britain's great country house estates and it's on our doorstep. It's a fine neo-classical mansion set in 50 acres of gardens.

The gardens are beautiful but not a major attraction for toddlers. Where Tatton comes into its own for the under-fives is in what surrounds the house and garden. Its 1,000-acre parkland is home to deer, cattle and sheep and boasts a rare breeds farm, an adventure playground and even a land train. Tatton also hosts a heap of special events throughout the year. The day we went there was a selection of small fairground rides.

We left the car in one of the huge fields dedicated to parking and decided to stroll to the farm as it didn't look too daunting for our three-year-old. This is a beautiful traditional farm with all you'd expect (see Home Farm on page 34).

We took the land train back to the main estate, stopping at the Stables Restaurant for lunch (the toilet block in the courtyard has baby changing facilities). From there, it was fairground rides all the way to the adventure playground. We found this exceptional. Containing over 30 rides, your toddler would happily have you here all day. It's a massive space set in beautiful surroundings and has been very well thought out.

Tatton Park's a really big deal. It's dominated this part of Cheshire for over two centuries and is, quite literally, a national treasure. If you don't fancy any of the above, just explore the park by foot, bike or even horse. You can park up for nothing in Knutsford and wander in with your buggies. With its woodland, ponds and lakes, this is a stunningly beautiful estate.

Low Season: Up to March 27th 2009 and Oct 5th 2009-March 26th 2010
Park: Tues-Sun 11am-5pm; Gardens, Shops and Restaurant: Tues-Sun 11am-4pm; Farm: Weekends 11am-4pm; Mansion: Closed except Oct 27th-Nov 1st and Christmas.
High Season: March 28th 2009-Oct 4th 2009
Park: Mon-Sun 10am-7pm; Gardens: Tues-Sun 10am-6pm; Mansion: Tues-Sun 1-5pm; Farm: Tues-Sun 12-5pm; Shops: Tues-Sun 10.30am-5pm; Restaurant: Mon-Sun 10am-6pm.
Last admission one hour before closing.
Park entry is £4.50 per car, free to walkers and cyclists. Up to March 27th 2009 Adult £4, Child £2, Family £10; Totally Tatton ticket (entry to 3 attractions) Adult £6, Child £3, Under 4s free, Family £15.
March 28th 2009-March 26th 2010 Adult £4.50, Child £2.50, Under 4s free, Family £11.50
Totally Tatton ticket (entry to 3 attractions) Adult £7, Child £3.50, Under 4s free, Family £11.50.
Tatton Park, Knutsford, Cheshire WA16 6QN
Tel: 01625 374400 www.tattonpark.org.uk.
Train to: Knutsford.

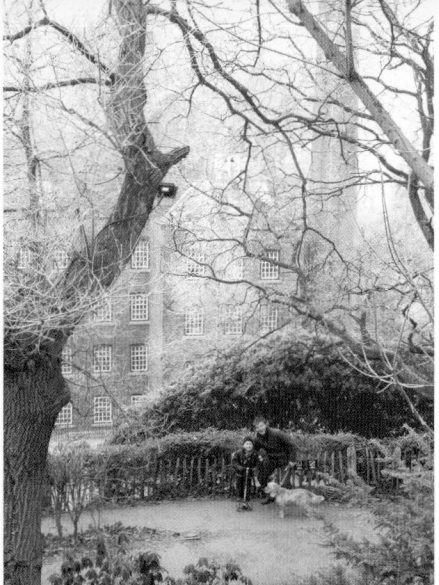

Both inside and outside Quarry Bank Mill is impressive. When the machines are running, the volume is incredible.

incredible. The rooms are big open spaces so it is easy to let kids run a bit wild. When you reach the bottom of the mill, there is a spectacular water wheel, the most powerful in Europe.

The Apprentice House is a guided tour that is booked in time slots and has limited availability. It is aimed at older children as the tour involves how the Victorian children used to live, where they slept, and even a vegetable garden. The Secret Garden was opened last year and although beautiful, is a bit tricky with pushchairs as it's built on a slope. Beware: there is also a river at the bottom so don't let children wander too far.

The restaurant is child friendly, offering lunch boxes at £2.95 or a child's meal at £3.50 for food such as sausage and mash or a Sunday lunch half portion at £3.95. No baby food is provided but they are happy to microwave food and bottles. There is a small play area in the corner and high chairs are available.

Mill: Mon-Sun 28th Feb-31st Oct 11am-5pm, Wed-Sun 1st Nov-28th Feb 2010 11am-4pm.
Apprentice House: timed tours. Estate open all year 7am-6pm. Last admission one hour before closing.
Mill: Adult £7, Child £3.70. Family ticket £17.70.
Estate: £4 per car.
Mill and Garden or Apprentice House: Adult £10, Child £5, Family ticket £24.
Mill, Garden and Apprentice House: Adult £13.50, Child £6.70, Family ticket £33.70.
Discounted combined rail, bus and entry tickets – enquire at your local station.
Quarry Bank Mill and Styal Estate (National Trust Property), Styal, Wilmslow, Cheshire SK9 4LA.
Tel: 01625 445896 www.nationaltrust.org.uk
Bus to: Quarry Bank Mill entrance (200). Train to: Styal, then walk.

Attractions and theme parks

Whether it's digging with giant JCBs, riding the Troublesome Trucks rollercoaster or simply stripping down and walking barefoot in a mudbath, this is a selection of hand-picked trips out of the city to suit everyone's tastes.

Attractions and theme parks

Apple Jacks Farm

Having received a very enthusiastic recommendation about Apple Jacks Farm, I was keen to road test it. We visited in October half term – on a particularly chilly day when the park had transformed itself into Spooky World. Unfortunately we chose the busiest time of day to arrive and with only one out of three ticket booths open, the queue to get in took more than 40 minutes. In fairness, they did open a second booth but it was a little too late for us.

We had packed a picnic and so, to revive ourselves, we headed straight to the covered eating area, where you can eat both food bought at the park and from home, which makes a refreshing change. We sat at a table with another family who had ordered from the self-service outdoor café, and despite complaining of a long wait to be served, they said their food was really nice and reasonably priced. The menu included options such as barbecued sausage hotdogs and jacket potatoes with beans and salad. On the good side, it was not a problem to warm baby food. And even better, there was a dance stage in the eating area and music playing, which the children loved.

The next stop was pig racing, which we enjoyed from the safety of a small grandstand at the side of the racetrack. Then it was on to the haunted house, which is a seasonal feature. Had it been a little warmer we probably would have given this a miss considering the young age of our children (one and four) but because of the cold we decided to take advantage of the opportunity to head indoors. The scary actors were gracious enough not to jump out on us – they reserved that pleasure for a group of teenagers following hot on our tail. All in all it was a good experience.

Other key features include go-karts, a giant bouncy pillow, a straw bale castle, and a sand pit complete with mini diggers. There are the added attractions of animals (Apple Jacks is a working farm), tractor rides and a maize maze. My only tip would be for those with very young children to visit during the warmer months as there is very little available indoors.

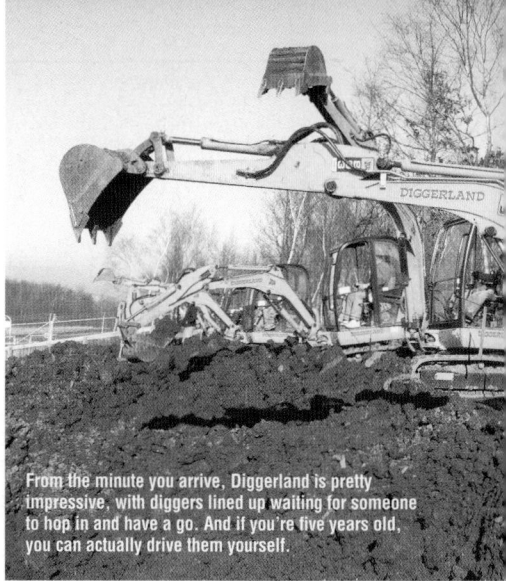

From the minute you arrive, Diggerland is pretty impressive, with diggers lined up waiting for someone to hop in and have a go. And if you're five years old, you can actually drive them yourself.

The park is easily accessible by pram, with purpose-built paths throughout. Baby changing facilities are only available in the ladies' toilets but as these are within a raised portakabin, prams have to be left outside.

At the time of going to press, prices and times for 2009 were not yet available but the park is generally open most weekends and school holidays throughout the year (2008 price for a family of four £34). Card payments incur a 40p charge.

Apple Jacks Farm, Stretton Road, Stretton, Warrington WA4 4NW Tel: 01925 268495
www.applejacksfarm.co.uk

Diggerland

We had friends visiting and when you're faced with five children ranging in age from two to nine years old, it can be tricky finding somewhere with something for everyone, but Diggerland is definitely a strong contender. The entrance fee, is fairly steep at £15 per person. Children under the age of three do go free but unfortunately there's no family ticket available. However, you can book online and save £2 per person, which is well worth doing. Or take advantage of our fantastic promotion on page 95 – a voucher offering two for one entry!

From the minute you arrive, Diggerland is pretty impressive – there are JCBs lined up on either side of the park just waiting for someone to hop in and have a go. They are all static but you can move the arm and bucket around and there are loads of levers to play with. A good place to start is to your left, which is where the Mini Diggers are situated. There are 12 of them, all of which do different activities

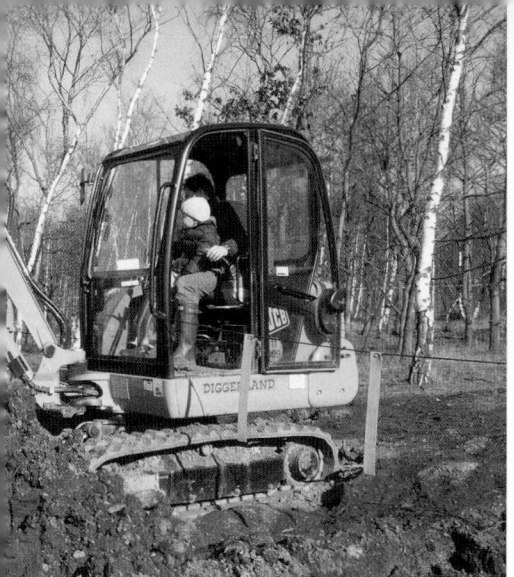

with buckets instead of seats. There are also coin-operated dodgems, which of course they all wanted a go on. And for the little ones, we discovered an indoor soft play area, which was another big hit.

New in 2008 was Joyrider – a Mitsubishi Pajero, done up to look like a police car which, from nine years old, you can have a go at driving around a track, complete with a marshal in the passenger seat and three passengers in the back, if they dare!

We went in the winter months and it was very quiet, but other mums who have been in the summer holidays said the longest wait they had was only 10 minutes, so a definite thumbs up on that front.

For children mad about diggers, Diggerland is a fantastic treat.

Weekends and daily during school holidays
Mar-Oct 10am-5pm, Nov-Feb 10am-4pm.
Admission: 3-65 yrs £15, Under 3s free.
Pre-booked on-line tickets £2 discount.
Diggerland, Willowbridge Lane, Whitwood, Castleford, West Yorkshire WF10 5NW
Tel: 0871 22 77 007 www.diggerland.com

Gulliver's World

Gulliver's is a theme park designed for families with children between the age of two and 13. Parts of it were beginning to look a bit tired, but there were plenty of new attractions and it sounds like there is a lot of investment planned for 2009.

We went during term time so it was pleasantly quiet. I understand from fellow mums that it does get busy in the summer holidays but not as bad as a lot of other theme parks. I would definitely recommend taking a pushchair as Gulliver's is vast. If you do forget though, buggies can be hired for £3 per day from guest services, which is on your right after the entrance before the bridge. Also available here are nappies and dummies plus you can pick up a sticker for your child to wear with your mobile number on, so that if they wander off, staff can easily contact you. (In truth, I tend to write my number on the backs of my children's hands with a pen when we're on day trips of this nature.)

Gulliver's is made up of themed areas and within each of these you will find a ride to suit your child's age. In particular, we enjoyed the train ride, which takes you around The Lost World; the pedal tractor driving school; and the mechanical diggers, which can be used to scoop up piles of plastic balls. These rides are all free. We also spent a lot of time in the Castle Play area, which is basically a playground, and found Western World was good for little ones as it had a fort they could run around on, a plane ride and the Pony Express – a horse on a carousel going round a track. Circus World was another feature that was particularly good for the younger children, with a ladybird and toy town ride.

with their buckets – knock down skittles, dig up bricks or pick up ducks. The five year olds can have a go on their own but younger children need to ride with an adult. Opposite the Mini Diggers are their Giant counterparts – three enormous diggers sitting on big piles of mud, which can be used to dig holes or just move earth around from one pile to another.

In the centre of the park are three areas: the first contains dumper trucks; the second, skid steers that go really slowly but are difficult to manoeuvre; and finally the tractors, which are extremely quick, and probably my favourite as you can get four in a car. Again you have to be five years old to drive but only three to go on all of the rides.

The café is still being built and should hopefully be ready by Easter 2009. In the meantime, take a picnic – when we went the only alternative was a burger van, though at least you could get a cup of tea. There are plenty of picnic tables outside and some available inside. Baby changing facilities are by the main building.

Other attractions at the park are go-karts for older children; the Sky Shuttle – where you sit in seats in the bucket of a digger and are transported 50 feet into the air, where the views are fantastic; and lastly Spin Dizzy – an enormous digger with eight seats in its bucket which as the name suggests, spins you round and round and bounces you up and down until you literally plead to get off! The older children loved it, but all the adults looked green. Both these rides are for three years and over but I really would think twice about letting your three year old on Spin Dizzy. For a more sedate time, try either the tractor that pulls a long line of trailers slowly around the park, or Dig-a-round – a carousel

Attractions and theme parks

Gulliver's also has an indoor centre with soft play, a kids' gym, which is basically a scaled down version of what you'll find in most private gyms, and face painting, which cost £3.50.

We'd brought a picnic and ate at one of the tables that are scattered throughout the park. The food on sale tended to be fast food style with chicken burger, chips and a drink for £2.50, but they also had packed lunches for the same price, which comprised a cheese roll, crisps, fruit, a chocolate biscuit and a drink.

One thing to bear in mind is that I made the mistake of going on my own with my two boys, Sam aged two and Harry, four. Whilst Harry was old enough to go on most of the rides (and had paid full price for the privilege), the fact that he was under 120cm high meant he had to be accompanied on the bigger ones. Unfortunately Sam was too small to come with us and of course couldn't be left unsupervised, so Harry had to miss out on quite a few rides. A word of advice: if you have children of mixed ages, make sure there's more than one adult.

As we were going to press, two new sections at Gulliver's were under construction. The first will be a sort of village-style play area (due to be ready by February 2009 half-term) with a mini shop, post office and interactive cooking area. The second, due to open by Easter, is an indoor water-themed area.
Feb half term 10.30am-5.30pm, Mon-Sun 4th Apr-30th Sep 10.30am-5.30pm, Sat and Sun 1st Oct-8th Nov 10.30am-5.30pm, Thurs-Sun Dec 10.30am-5.30pm. Admission: Adults and children £12.50, children under 90cm free.
Gulliver's Theme Park Warrington, Old Hall, Warrington WA5 9YZ
Tel: 01925 444888 www.gulliversfun.co.uk

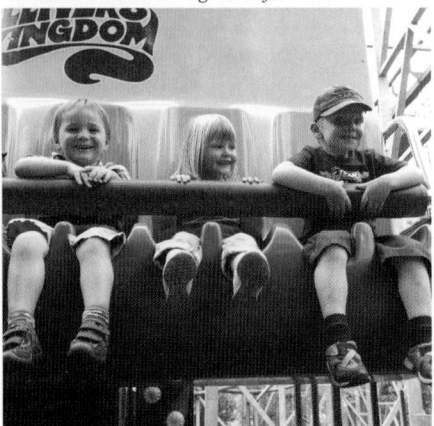

Gulliver's is aimed at families with children aged between two and 13. It is made up of themed areas and within each of these you will find a ride to suit your child's age.

Red House Farm

I've been struggling with quite how to sum up Red House Farm to the uninitiated. So I'll cheat and say it's a bit of everything – you've got a farm shop serving up wonderful fresh produce and regional specialities; award-winning tea rooms dishing out delicious doorstopper sandwiches and tempting cakes; an outdoor area with sandpit and motorised mini vehicles; and in the summertime a Maize Maze with a barbecue, bouncy castle, pedal quad bikes, play area, and a quad barrel train.

I took my two year old and his Granny there in the summer. We started with lunch at the outside tables in the cobbled courtyard area. We all opted for sandwiches – there is a good children's menu with things like the picnic platter (ham, cheese, crisps, fruit and bread) for £3.95 or they also offer dishes from the organic 'Baby Deli' range which start at £2. The staff were very helpful (they will happily heat up baby bottles etc) and the food arrived quickly and was tasty. Whilst Granny and I slugged the remains of our drinks, Will took himself off to the little play area which is just in view of the tea rooms. He pottered in the sand pit for a bit, then insisted we help put him on the motorised mini-diggers and tractors (£1 coin operated so bring some change!)

After this, a short walk away from the tea rooms in the summer months is the 'Redhouse Farm Maize Maze', set up on one of the top fields. You have to pay to get in but there are lots of activities as well as a spectacular looking maize. We started with the bouncy castle then once he'd tired of that, we headed for the quad barrel train. Granny and Will squeezed themselves into a blue plastic oil-drum type thing (Will was too young to ride on his own) and off they zoomed, with around eight other barrels behind a noisy quad bike, round a cornfield. They returned about five minutes later a bit muddy and definitely windswept – Will seemed to enjoy himself though not sure about Granny!

The giant sandpit with various toys in it kept Will entertained for the longest amount of time – he also played on the straw mountain a bit and in the Little Tikes play area but that was about his limit. We finished off with an ice cream (all refreshments cost extra) and headed home. The only disappointment for Will was the fact that apart from some rabbits and guinea pigs there were no large farm animals – so be prepared to talk your way out of that one!

Baby changing facilities are in the unisex toilets next to the tea rooms. Car parking is free.
Tea rooms open Mon-Sat 9am-4.30pm, Sun 10am-4.30pm; Farm shop open Mon-Sat 9am-5.30pm, Sun 10am-4.30pm; Maize open July-Sept.

OUT AND ABOUT

Admission: Adult £5.95, Child £4.95, Under 5s free.
Party of four (regardless of adult:child ratio) £19.50.
Redhouse Farm, Redhouse Lane, Dunham Massey,
Altrincham WA14 5RL
Tel: 0161 941 3480 www.redhousefarm.co.uk
Bus to: Sinderland Lane (247, from Altrincham Interchange).
Tram to: Altrincham, then bus. Train to: Altrincham, then bus.

Thomas Land

We're two, we're four, we're six, we're eight, shunting trains and hauling freight... Well, if you're going to brave a theme park with little ones, you might as well embrace it! A trip to Thomas Land at Drayton Manor Theme Park had been on our agenda for quite a while – but we had to work it out with almost military precision. We'd been warned by other parents who'd gone on a Bank Holiday weekend that the queues had been horrific, so we definitely wanted to go on a term time weekday as we were hoping this would be a little quieter and cheaper. A good tip is that reduced price adult-toddler tickets are available mid-week during Staffordshire term times (these times may differ from Manchester). We set off at 10am from Manchester and found ourselves pulling into the car park around 11.30am, nice and easy so far. There is lots of parking as you'd expect and we were able to park pretty close to the entrance. It took us about five minutes to walk to the main ticket area.

Once in, we headed straight to Thomas Land, which is an attraction within Drayton Manor immediately on your left-hand side after walking through the gates. We spotted 'Harold's Heli Tours' (Harold the Helicopter takes you round in a circle then up into the sky) and headed straight for it. Unfortunately we had to queue for around 40 minutes to get on and it didn't even look that busy! We had to remind ourselves that the kids were enjoying it but adult spirits were definitely beginning to ebb at this point as we were expecting every queue to be a similar length. However, by around 12.30pm it all seemed to quieten down. Whether this was because people were having lunch or had arrived earlier than us and moved onto another part of the park we never discovered. But whatever it was, the queues were a lot faster moving after that.

There are 12 themed rides to go on. These include the Troublesome Trucks runaway coaster – a 220m roller coaster that runs up and over Thomas Land; Rockin' Bulstrode and Sodor Docks – a bumpy ride that rotates you 360 degrees; and Sodor's classic cars, where you steer a car through tunnels and a barn. Our children were aged two and three and in my opinion a little young for some of the rides. Bear in mind as well that generally you need one adult to accompany each child on a ride.

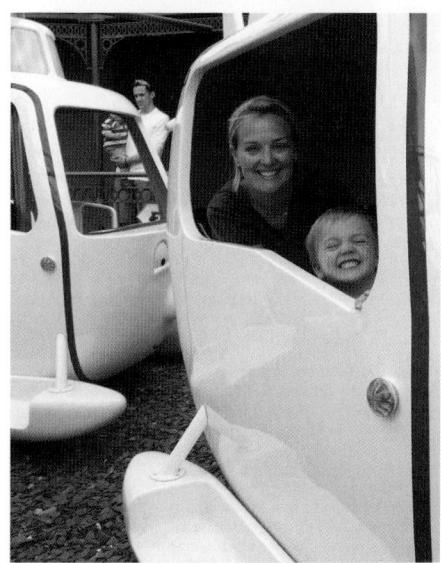

There are 12 themed rides to go on at Thomas Land, including the Troublesome Trucks runaway coaster, Rockin' Bulstrode and Sodor Docks.

After some good Thomas adventures we decided to have lunch. We'd brought our own picnic but trying to find somewhere to eat it in the Thomas Land section was tricky as the few benches were all full. We finally got lucky and all squashed up together. We discovered later that there are plenty more (outdoor) picnic areas in the zoo section, which isn't far away, so next time we'd probably factor that in and head there. There is a café in the Thomas area, one of several throughout the park. They stock Ella's organic range of food pouches for babies and toddlers, which we thought was very good.

Lunch break over, we climbed aboard Percy the train for a gentle ride out of Thomas Land to Farmer McColls Farm, where there's a café, an exotic animal reserve and what our children wanted most – Spencer's Activity Park. This is a brilliant, large adventure playground with tonnes of equipment for the kids to run amok on. After the best part of an hour we managed to drag the children off and ambled back towards the entrance via the zoo. We didn't get round all of it but we saw tigers, monkeys and penguins, among others, so we felt like we were getting our money's worth.

We finished off with Emily's Adventure Play – a large indoor soft play area situated to the side of Thomas Land. We thought it was excellent – the play is controlled on a time basis so it was never over-crowded. No adults were allowed in the play zone (but there were comfy sofas for you to relax

Attractions and theme parks

on) – it was controlled by a staff member who made sure all the children were ok, although this could be tricky if your children are clingy. There is also a good area for under twos and baby changing on site.

There are toilets and baby changing in Thomas Land and the zoo section (in total there are six baby changing facilities and three mother and baby feeding areas around the park) but some could definitely do with a facelift and could have been cleaner.

Overall, we all had a great day out – totally exhausting but the children loved every minute of it.
Sat 21st March 2009-Sun 1st Nov 2009.
The whole park is closed on selected days in Sep and Oct. During the Christmas period Drayton Manor will be closed but Thomas Land will open at a reduced price. Gates open at 9.30am and rides start at 10.30am and close at either 5pm or 6pm, depending on the time of year.
2008 prices Adult £23, Child £19, Under 4s free, Adult and Toddler (under 4 years) available only during Staffordshire term time £14.
Discounts available by booking on line.
Thomas Land at Drayton Manor Theme Park, Tamworth, Staffordshire B78 3TW
Tel: 0844 472 1960 www.draytonmanor.co.uk
© 2009 Gullane (Thomas) Limited.

Trentham Gardens and Adventure Play – Barfuss Park (Barefoot Walk)

We were recommended Trentham Gardens and the Barefoot Walk by a friend who loved it. The only time I'd really seen or heard about it was on one of the brown signs off the M6, so I was quite intrigued.

We arrived to be greeted by a row of shops and a large restaurant, not overly impressed so far... After locating the entrance, right in the centre of the actually very nice independent shopping village, we headed into the gardens, where we were rewarded with the sight of the beautiful Italian gardens and an enormous lake.

We headed straight over to the Adventure Play Area, where there is a rather brilliant choice of three play areas, two large sandpits full of toys, diggers

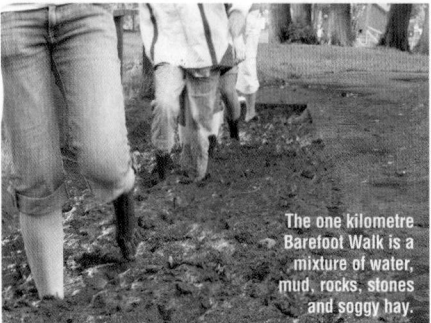

The one kilometre Barefoot Walk is a mixture of water, mud, rocks, stones and soggy hay.

and wheelbarrows and the JCB track – a tarmac pathway with at least 10 pedal diggers in various sizes. The play areas are aimed at different ages and abilities, the first one from 18 months, the second from three years and the third from eight upwards. What I loved about it most though were the numerous deckchairs and picnic tables scattered around. Although not the sunniest day, it was great to just plonk down, admire the view and watch my sons amuse themselves. Totally relaxing. Not something that's ever happened on a family day trip before!

At last I managed to rouse myself and tear everyone away from the play area to attempt the one kilometre Barefoot Walk (Barfuss Park in German). After storing shoes and bags in the lockers provided, we set off across water, mud, rocks, stones and soggy hay. Strangely enough, the boys took a bit of persuading to wade through the mud – I couldn't believe that my rough and tumble two-year-old flatly refused to step in it – but we eventually made it round. Foot showers are provided at the end of the walk, although the mud does take a bit of washing off.

We'd brought a picnic, which was a good job as the café was in the process of being demolished! A new site is being built, which should be open by Easter 2009, and will contain new toilets with baby changing facilities. There will be a temporary marquee serving hot drinks and pre-packed food but there are plenty of places to eat in the shopping village. Until the new café is built there are no baby changing facilities within the gardens. However, there are two baby changing toilets in the village and there is no problem going in and out of the park.

The lake and woodlands are found immediately on your right as you come out of the gardens. Here you'll find The Fern Miniature Railway, a narrow gauge train that runs along the shore of the lake at £2 per person. There is also a 42-seat catamaran, Miss Elizabeth, that cruises the lake for £2.50 per person or you can hire your own rowing boats for £7 per family. There are various walks round the Trentham Estate, two of which are pushchair friendly. The Lakeside Café only serves hot drinks and pre-packed food but staff are happy to provide hot water for heating bottles and baby food.
Trentham Gardens and Adventure Play: 1st Oct-31st Mar 10am-4pm, 1st Apr-30th Sep 10am-6pm.
Winter 2008: Adult £5, Child 5-15 £2.50, Under 5s free. Family ticket £15. Summer 2009: Adult £7, Child 3-15 £6, Under 3s free. Family ticket £24.
Trentham Woodlands and Lake: 8am-8pm or one hour before dusk. Admission free. For operating times of the train and the boat please see website.
The Trentham Estate, Stone Road, Trentham, Stoke-on-Trent, Staffordshire ST4 8AX
Tel: 01782 646646 www.trenthamleisure.co.uk

Greater Manchester may well be land-locked but fortunately it is within a stone's throw of the west coast of England, which has a great selection of beaches – perfect for day trips.

"Manchester's got everything except a beach"

Ian Brown, Stone Roses.

Formby Point Red Squirrel Reserve

This reserve is National Trust owned and includes a pine forest squirrel reserve and Formby Sands. This is uncommercialised stunning natural coast without a pier or prom in sight. If you're heading to the squirrel reserve first then park under the trees, but if you are intending to take a Crackerjack-worthy collection of items onto the beach then it is better to park a little closer and walk back to the squirrels unladen.

A short hike over grass-covered sand dunes from the car park took us to the wild open beach of Formby Sands. The dunes were great for 'sand sliding' and the firm sand was equally as good for football as it was for making sand-castles. In some places there was clay on the beach, which was slippy and squelchy, but my children and their friends found it brilliant fun. With its exposed position, kite flying is popular, but the wind ate its way into everything, so be prepared for sand-sandwiches!

Even with a three-wheeler it is diffi-cult to push a pram over the sand dunes but the squirrel reserve is very pram-friendly. The reserve borders the dunes and is home to one of the UK's last remaining colonies of red squirrels. You can purchase bags of nuts at the entrance lodge to encourage the squir-rels down from the trees. On a visit a couple of years ago we saw several but on this recent trip we saw far less as sadly squirrel pox has reduced their numbers. There are toilets next to the reserve but they are some distance from the beach. On a warm day there is an ice-cream van but nowhere else to purchase refreshments, so pack a picnic.
All year dawn until dusk. Toilets close summer 5.30pm, winter 4pm. Admission: £3 car entry.
Formby Point Red Squirrel Reserve, Victoria Road, Freshfield, Formby, Liverpool L37 1LJ
Tel: 01704 878591 www.nationaltrust.org.uk

St Annes

St Annes is a much smaller, quieter beach resort than neighbouring Blackpool but still has the pier and promenade, with all the attractions that young children love at the seaside. A day trip here is a regular occurrence in our household.

We usually park in the pay and display car park by the

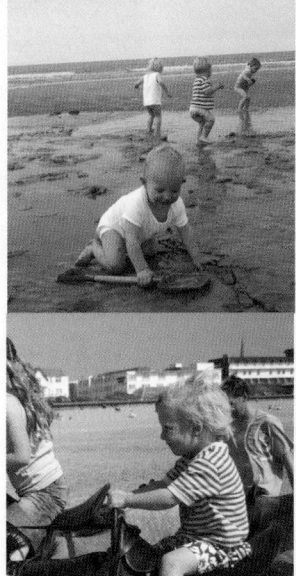

Formby Point Red Squirrel Reserve and St Annes are two of the area's top beach destinations.

Beach Terrace, a lovely stand-alone café with great views about 500m south of the pier – ideal for a quick cup of tea before you start. Baby changing and high chairs are available. Then we head north along the prom towards the pier – often the boys take their bikes, as it is an ideal surface to cycle on and they can get to the attractions a bit quicker. Spoilt for choice they begin on their favourite, the little train, which takes a circular route round the crazy golf taking in a tunnel along the way. From there it's on to the netted trampolines. There are a number of other attractions including boats and a bouncy play area in close proximity, all suitable for children under five.

The pier is a little bit tired but full of the type of little rides that small children adore. Most of the rides and attractions are open from Easter until the October half-term. The costs vary, but are in the region of £1.50 and generally cash only.

The beach itself is beautiful, and on the north side of the pier it is bordered by sand dunes which can either be explored or used as shelter from the wind. During the summer months, the tide is low during the main part of the day, so it is a long walk to the sea, but we usually manage it, collecting washed up shells and seaweed in a bucket on the way. If the walk seems a bit too far, there is a purpose-built paddling pool for toddlers on the promenade, close to the pier, for a splash.

There is also a café on the pier, unsurprisingly called the Pier Café, and adjacent to that a fish and chip shop. For lunch however we either return to the Beach Terrace Café or more commonly pack a picnic and eat it sat in the sand dunes. After lunch we make sandcastles on the beach before the boys are lured to the donkeys and the inflatable bouncy slide. Exhausted from all the fun they always fall asleep within five minutes of leaving St Annes.
Beach Terrace Café: Mon-Sun 9am-4pm, Closed Christmas Day and for two or three weeks in January.
Inner Promenade Junction, Fairhaven Road, St Annes FY8 1NN Tel: 01253 711167
Pier Café: Mon-Sun Easter-31st Oct 10am-6pm, Sat and Sun 1st Nov-Easter 10am-4pm.
The Pier Café, St Annes Pier, South Promenade, St Annes FY8 2NG Tel: 01253 788510 or 07834 452899 www.piercafe.co.uk

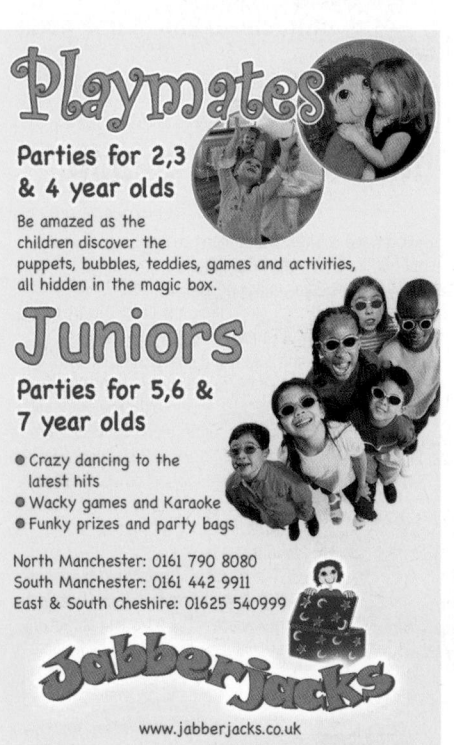
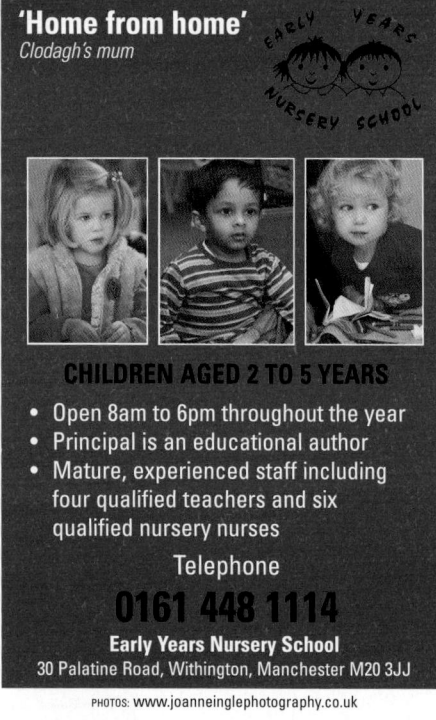
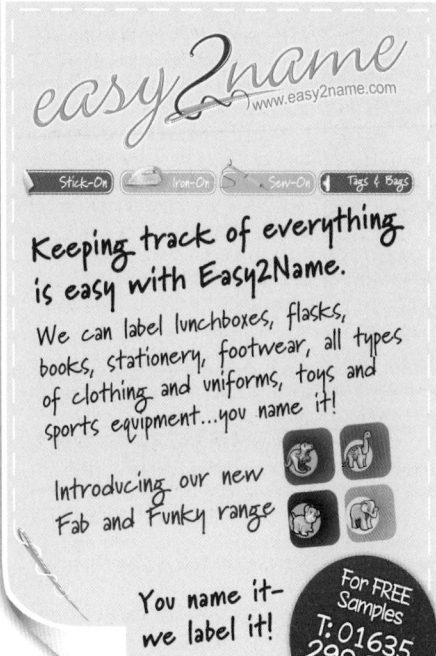

Manchester's restaurant scene is vibrant and varied. From Greek to Italian; French to Indonesian, our list offers a child-friendly introduction to just about every type of food. Each restaurant we've reviewed has baby changing, highchairs and will happily heat up bottles and baby food unless stated otherwise.

Eating out

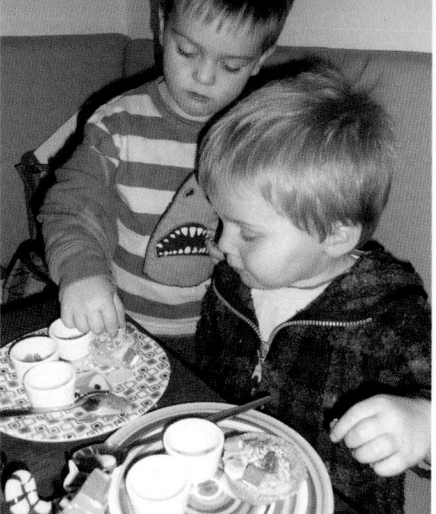

Cup cake decorating at Queenie Mumbles.

Barburrito

Because I love Mexican food, I'd been really looking forward to trying out Barburrito with three year old Will. We went with his friend Toby and baby Daniel to the restaurant in the Trafford Centre. It was pretty quiet when we arrived at 12pm as they had only just opened.

The concept is basically fast-food style – order your dish at the counter and they'll prepare it freshly in front of you – pay, grab a drink and sit yourselves back down again. There is a "Mini Mex" menu for children. Priced at £3.95 you choose a small version of any of the adult choices and you get tortilla chips plus a soft drink (fizzy or water).

The children enjoyed watching the staff make up their meal. They shared a chicken quesadillas which was plenty big enough when supplemented with the free nachos. Mums shared a burrito and it was heavenly! The boys really tucked in well – loving the nachos of course.

For me it was a perfect lunch – tasty, healthy food and ready quickly. The restaurant doesn't have activity packs or any child diversions but because you're not waiting around for your food, it really doesn't matter. There was a lot of room next to the table, so parking the buggy with Daniel was easy.

There is another Barburrito in Piccadilly Gardens in Manchester city centre which we tried on a weekday lunchtime – it was very busy with professionals and I would recommend going to the Trafford Centre restaurant if you're taking children! Also check out their website before you go as there are regular offers.
Mon-Fri 11.30am-11pm, Sat 11am-11pm,
Sun 12noon-10pm
Barburrito, 134 The Orient, The Trafford Centre,
Manchester M17 8EH
Tel: 0161 747 6165 www.barburrito.co.uk
Also in Piccadilly Gardens, Manchester

Battery Park Juice Bar

A well-known institution amongst Chorlton-ites, we decided to give Battery Park a go with the kids in tow. Four of us went on a weekday for lunch – weekends do get very busy apparently – there is no children's menu so we decided on a cream cheese topped toasted bagel and a couple of hot halloumi sandwiches to share amongst us all. We split one milkshake between the children (they're enormous and very thick and did I mention delicious?!) and we settled for juices – the bill came to £18.35.

It's got a lovely atmosphere, a real community vibe – the café's split-level with wooden chairs and tables downstairs and a couple of comfy sofas in the back room upstairs. We took along a bag of toy cars and our two kept themselves entertained enough for lunch not to be too stressful. They have a highchair but there is no baby changing facilities.

Quite frankly it's not brilliantly child friendly and you'd struggle to get pushchairs in when it's busy but if you're passing, fancy a brilliant smoothie or chunky sandwich, it's definitely worth a look.
Mon-Fri 8am-5.30pm, Sat 10am-6pm, Sun 11am-5pm
Battery Park Juice Bar, 615a Wilbraham Road,
Chorlton M21 9AN Tel: 0161 860 0754

Brasserie Chez Gerard

We really put Chez Gerard to the test…it was Saturday teatime in mid-December with the Christmas Market across the road and absolutely heaving with people. I don't think I've ever seen Manchester city centre busier. We fought our way to the door and asked if they had a table for three; we hadn't booked. The manager hesitated for just a moment before racking his brains and smiling 'yes, but only for an hour or so'. He led us through the throng and reset a table that had already been laid out for a Christmas party.

Despite our son being in a terrible mood, the staff were terrific and couldn't do enough for him. We asked for an activity pack but were told they'd all gone – it had been their busiest day of the year.

Restaurants

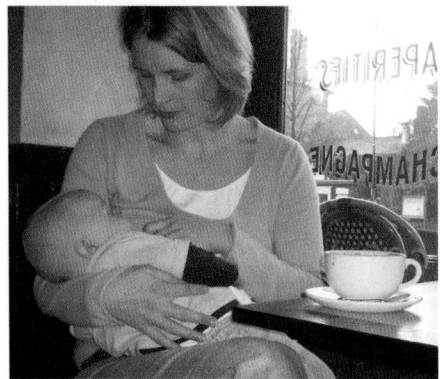

At Café Rouge on a week day it is usually pleasantly quiet. So a collection of novice pram drivers pushing all our vehicles in with their precious cargo didn't feel so intimidated!

Nevertheless, the waitress was soon to be seen on hands and knees, scrambling around locating lost crayons to colour in the children's menu. It was good value; a basket of baguette with butter, a main course, soft drink and a dessert for £5.95. Main choices were chicken with new potatoes, fish and chips, hamburger and chips, penne pasta and a cheese or plain omelette. The choice of dessert was impressive too. Ice creams and sorbets, fresh fruit, mixed grapes and a Belgian waffle with hot chocolate sauce.

This is a good choice for a family meal in the city centre. Adult food is tasty and the staff really couldn't have been better. *Mon-Thurs 10am-10pm, Fri-Sat 10am-11pm, Sun 11am-10pm Brasserie Chez Gerard, 2-8 Commercial Union House, Albert Square, Manchester M2 6LW Tel: 0161 834 7633 www.brasseriechezgerard.co.uk*

Café Rouge

Café Rouge was a winning choice for me when I wanted to meet up with fellow new mums and our babies. We used to meet regularly mid-morning, post one feed and pre-another, nervously discussing in the most intricate detail the sleeping patterns of our respective newborns over a hot chocolate and a croissant.

The thing I liked most about Café Rouge was at this time of day it was usually pleasantly quiet. So a collection of novice pram drivers with our precious cargo didn't feel so intimidated!

I've since returned with my toddler and found the staff just as amenable and the children's menu is

TOP FIVE PLACES TO EAT
The Olive Press
The only restaurant we've found where toddlers under three eat free, brilliant!
Carluccio's
Delicious italian food with friendly staff – a great place to take kids.
Tampopo
Award winning family restaurant, this noodle bar and it's spicy crackers always hits the mark.
Queenie Mumbles
A lovely cafe prepared to go the extra mile for it's younger clientele! They'll cook anything the children want.
Barburrito
Fresh, wholesome and great fun for little fingers.

fairly priced with a good selection such as chicken, mash and gravy or cheesy omelette and fries, with dessert and drink for £4.95. Most branches have step free access and outside seating. *Mon-Thurs and Sun 9am-11pm, Fri-Sat 9am-midnight Café Rouge, 651-653 Wilmslow Rd, Manchester M20 6QZ Tel: 0161 438 0444 www.caferouge.co.uk Also at The Trafford Centre and City Centre Manchester*

Carluccio's

An authentic Italian menu and a welcome relief from the throng of shoppers at the Trafford Centre! Going to Carluccio's for lunch was a complete treat – a perfect, delicious escape. The waiting staff fell over themselves to coo at the babies at another table and they expressed delight at everything my two year old did.

The children's menu at £5.95 was excellent with a good choice of dishes that included breadsticks and a soft drink to start, followed by pasta with different sauces, lasagne or ravioli, with smaller portions available off the main menu if nothing appealed. Lastly gorgeous ice cream, I was practically praying Sam wouldn't finish it – simply divine.

A great little activity pack kept the children entertained between courses and nothing was a problem for the staff. Baby facilities were on site – no traipsing to the other end of the Trafford Centre. I will definitely be heading back soon. *Mon-Sat 9am-12midnight, Sun 10am-12midnight Carluccio's, The Great Hall, The Trafford Centre, Manchester M17 8AA Tel: 0161 747 4973 www.carluccios.com Also at Spinningfields*

Coriander Restaurant

I never would have thought a year ago when I started this project that I would be able to go for a curry on a Friday night with children. But amazingly that's what happened and both boys were brilliant. We didn't start our night aiming for a curry but that's where we ended up at an usually late hour of 7.30pm. The restaurant was pretty busy and full by the time we left. We quickly ordered poppadoms and even got the boys trying the dips. While I was glancing through the menu it was only after a few minutes that I realised it was the children's menu. It was a very extensive and varied list, priced around £7.90 for a main course, rice and chips including a drink or ice cream. We ordered one curry and let them share which was plenty.

There are no baby changing facilities or crayons, but the staff were very friendly and accommodating. They're more than happy to warm up milk and they do have highchairs.

Coriander uses all natural ingredients and has no added food colourings. I have to say both my husband's meal and mine were delicious. So curry with the kids? No problem.

Mon-Thurs 5.30-11.30pm, Fri and Sat 5.30-12pm, Sun 3-10pm
Coriander Restaurant, 279 Barlow Moor Road, Chorlton-cum-Hardy, Manchester M21 7GH
Tel: 0161 881 7750 www.coriandercholton.co.uk

Croma

Arriving at ten minutes to seven on a Thursday night to try out a different restaurant with two hungry and tired children I thought would be a recipe for disaster. The reality though was fantastic. I ordered their meal first and they had barely started colouring with the crayons provided when their pizzas arrived, our food wasn't far behind either.

The children's set menu is good value at £4.95, with a choice of drinks, pizza with ham or mushroom or tomato pasta and a delicious tub of Cheshire ice cream. The main menu choices were excellent and all at a reasonable price. It was full of young trendies out on the town as well as families, which made for a great atmosphere. Incredibly we were back home in Didsbury with both boys fast asleep by 8 o'clock, unlike the young trendies!

Baby changing facilities available but only in the ladies toilets.

Mon-Sat 12noon-11pm, Sun 12noon-10.30pm
Croma, 1-3 Clarence Street, Manchester M2 4DE
Tel: 0161 237 9799 www.croma.biz
Also at Chorlton and Prestwich

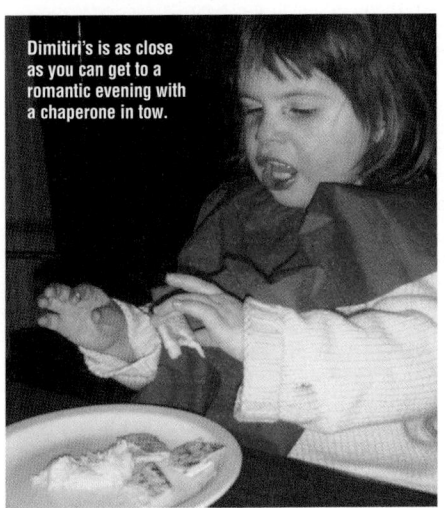
Dimitri's is as close as you can get to a romantic evening with a chaperone in tow.

Dimitri's

For me, the greek restaurant Dimitri's brings back memories of long leisurely evenings spent eating and drinking with friends – so I was a little apprehensive about allowing my two and a half year old to blow a hole in those rose tinted glasses ... but I need not have worried. It seems that even toddlers can be mood enhanced by a bit of chilled out lighting. Minutes later, hummus and pitta bread was having the same effect on her as San Miguel was having on us – soothing.

A main of pasta bolognese for her (okay so it's not exactly Greek, but anything for an easy life) and fish kebabs for us got serious thumbs up all around. The kids' bit of the menu has all the firm favourites – so even fussy eaters are well catered for. We had a lovely time – I'd say that this place is as close as you can get to a romantic evening when you've got a little chaperone in tow. The staff were really friendly too – they even told me I was a Pretty Princess – at least I think they were talking to me!?

Daily 11am-midnight
Dimitri's, Campfield Arcade, Tonman Street, Deansgate, Manchester M3 4FN
Tel: 0161 839 3319 www.dimitris.co.uk

Dukes 92

A favourite of ours pre-children, we decided to return to Dukes with our three year old in tow... For those who don't know it, Dukes 92 is located in a fabulous spot in the Castlefield area of central Manchester at the meeting point of the Bridgewater and Rochdale canals – in fact it takes its name from the adjacent Duke's Lock.

The pub-café interior is nice and spacious with a selection of booths or tables and chairs – it's all on the flat, so easy to get in with a buggy and park up next to your table. The canal side patio has plenty of seating too but of course being so close to the water's edge, you'd have to be vigilant with toddlers. Dukes specialises in pate & cheese (for the adults) as well as having sandwiches, salads and pizzas on offer. The kids' menu has four options – pizza, pasta, haddock goujons or chunky chicken all priced at £3.95. Drinks and desserts are extra. Will opted for the fish and it was a generous portion and very tasty.

All told we had a lovely time – it's not cheap, our bill came to £25 for three meals and soft drinks – but it's a perfect setting particularly on a sunny day.

Free parking in Dukes' car park next door or on the street in front.

Lunchtime menu Mon-Thurs 12noon-3pm;
Fri-Sun 12noon-4.30pm
Dukes 92, 18 Castle Street, Manchester M3 4LZ
Tel: 0161 839 8646 www.dukes92.com

EATING OUT

Restaurants

Frankie & Benny's

It's noisy, majorly child-friendly and the staff turn a complete blind eye as your little darlings make a right old mess in the leather booths. A UK wide chain, Frankie & Benny's offers a comprehensive children's menu with ten dishes to choose from, ranging from fish fingers to chicken pasta, all priced at £3.95 which includes unlimited soft drinks (not juice) and a dessert. There is also the option to ask for a free salad or vegetable side-order. A kids' activity pack is handed out on arrival and a balloon when you leave. The service when we went was extremely quick and they really couldn't do enough for the children. Baby-changing facilities were good and they offer free wipes and nappy bags on request.
Mon-Sat 10am-11pm, Sun 10am-10.30pm
Frankie & Benny's, 34 St. Annes Street, Manchester
M2 7LE Tel: 0161 835 2479
www.frankieandbennys.com
Frankie & Benny are located all over Greater Manchester so check website for details.

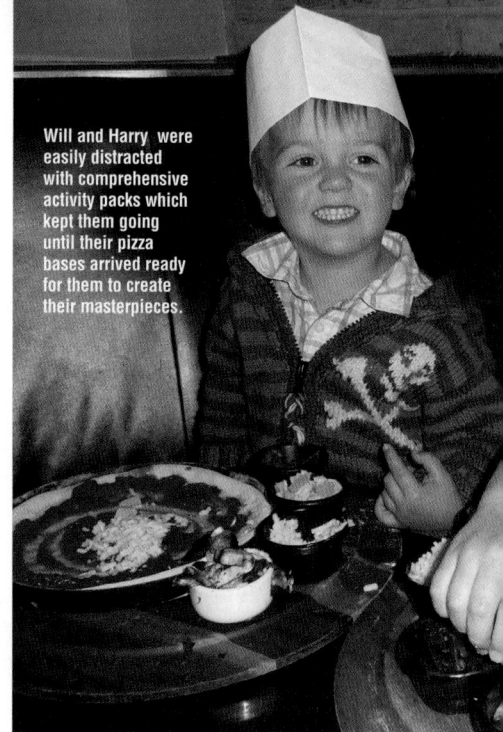

Will and Harry were easily distracted with comprehensive activity packs which kept them going until their pizza bases arrived ready for them to create their masterpieces.

Giraffe

Giraffe's got a reputation for being extremely family friendly. The intention of this chain is that their menus give customers "a flavour of the world," so if you've not been before, you'll find the food very varied indeed. For me, the adult choices were a bit overwhelming and quite expensive, but the children's menu is thankfully a little more simple. Our two chose crunchy chicken with fries and foccacia pizza fingers with salad and apple slices. Because we were there at lunchtime, we were able to go for the G-Kids Meal Deal which meant any children's main course plus dessert and drink was £5.75 (only available Mon-Fri till 4pm). Portions were generous and the food arrived promptly – as did the colouring pencils. Staff were very helpful and the boys were thrilled when they were given a balloon on their way out.
Mon-Fri 7.45am-11pm, Sat 9am-11pm, Sun 9am-10.30pm
Giraffe, Spinningfields Square, Deansgate, Manchester
M3 3AF Tel: 0161 839 0009 www.giraffe.net
Also at The Trafford Centre and Manchester Airport Terminal 1 Airside

Gourmet Burger Kitchen

The menu has a whopping 28 burgers to choose from with some very tasty twists on the classic burger. Gourmet Burger Kitchen is certainly child-friendly, there's a dedicated children's menu where they can order a burger (vegetarian option available), fries and drink for £5.85. Or there's the option to have chicken pieces instead for the same price. Our little boy wasn't perhaps quite at the age where he could get stuck into the food so it was a bit wasted on him. The food was delicious but there are no activity packs for little ones so take your own entertainment.

Sun-Thurs 12noon-10pm, Fri 12noon-11pm, Sat 11am-11pm
Gourmet Burger Kitchen, Spinningfields, Bridge Street, Manchester M3 3ER
Tel: 0161 832 2719 www.gbkinfo.com
Also at Didsbury and Wilmslow

Gusto

Gusto is a modern Italian restaurant offering more than just pasta and pizza. We arrived for an early lunch and although the waitress was very friendly and helpful, service was a bit slow and with three children it needed to be quicker. They were all easily distracted with pretty comprehensive activity packs and this kept them going until their pizza bases arrived ready for them to create their masterpieces. The cost was £5.95 for a pizza with a choice of various toppings, this also included dessert and a chef's hat. There is an alternative two course menu at £5.75 which included starters of calamari, garlic bread or ham and melon with a selection of pasta dishes for the main course. Drinks and dessert were extra though. Gusto stock the organic BabyDeli range which starts at £2.35 for a four month old baby puree meal.

For myself I ordered the penne pasta with salmon, peas and baby spinach and I think it's fair to say I had about three mouthfuls and the boys stole the rest, so I can honestly say the pizzas were good as that's what I ended up eating! There was no

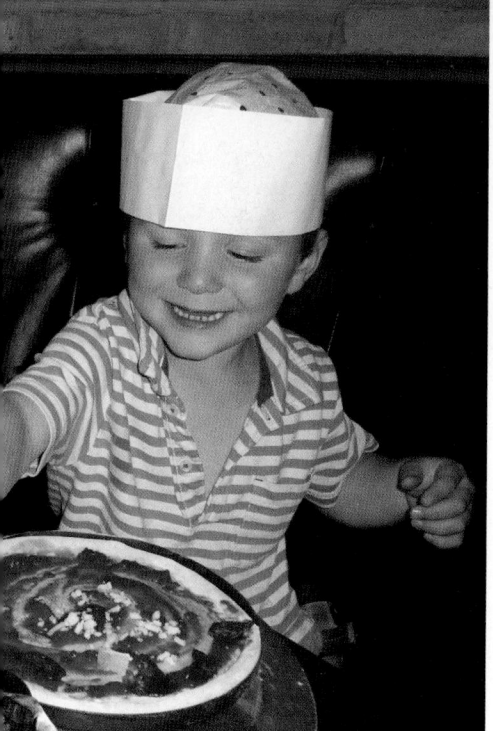

Jam Street Café

I'd only been to Jam Street Café in the evening for drinks and a spot of dinner, so thought it was worth a try in the name of research, to come back during the day with the kids. In the traditional sense they are not child friendly. There are no baby changing facilities, little room for pushchairs and no obvious children's menu. But, they do a great all day breakfast for £5.60 which is absolutely perfect to share with a little one or they are happy to go off piste and cook some beans on toast or something similar. Another children's favourite is the ice cream sundae or a babychino (warm frothy milk with chocolate sprinkle). Staff were lovely and didn't seem to mind too much when four mums with a child each took over the small café. They were more than willing to warm up a bottle of milk and grab a high chair from the basement. In the evening the café turns into a bar and food finishes around 9.30pm so children have to leave by then.
Sun-Thurs 10am-midnight, Fri-Sat 10am-1am
Jam Street Café, 209 Upper Chorlton Road, Whalley Range, Manchester M16 0BH Tel: 0161 881 9944

The Lead Station

An informal and popular cafe/bar where you can dine on three courses; take a leisurely breakfast or pop in for a coffee and cake. Housed in a former police station, The Lead Station always seems to be teeming with children of all ages (particularly around the early dinner slot of 6-8pm). This really helps to provide its informal and friendly atmosphere.

We are regulars, and Oliver my four year old, is so accustomed to the menu that he usually places his order as we are being shown to a table. My boys love it because the children's menu is good and the staff always take time to have a giggle with them. I love it because it is a night out in a trendy cafe bar. Some favourites on the menu are bangers and mash, steak, dips and pittas, and usually some delicious vegetarian options.

In summer there is a pleasant outdoor seating area to the rear. If you come armed with a pram, don't be put off by the three steep steps at the entrance and the swinging double entrance doors, once you get through this initial assault course it's plain sailing. Baby changing is on the first floor.
Mon-Weds 11am-9.30pm, Thurs-Fri 11am-10pm, Weekends 10am-10pm
The Lead Station, 99 Beech Road, Chorlton, Manchester M21 9EQ Tel: 0161 881 5559

Loch Fyne

I watched uncertainly as one of Didsbury's oldest establishments Ye Old Cock Inn was converted into a Loch Fyne fish restaurant. We went for lunch and there were quite a few families with children and

problem getting them all wrapped up to take away as we had loads left over. Two pizzas between three children would have been plenty.

After 6pm the children's menu stops and though they were happy to have children in the restaurant they could only provide a small version of the adult meals at a reduced rate.
Mon-Fri 11am-11pm, Weekends 10.30am-11pm.
The kitchen opens from 12noon.
Gusto, 756 Wilmslow Road, Didsbury M20 2DW
Tel: 0161 445 8209 www.gustorestaurants.uk.com
Also at Knutsford and Alderley Edge

Hullabaloo

We chanced upon this cute café on a shopping excursion to Altrincham with our eighteen month old boys. It's fully organic serving great tasting food including sandwiches, salads, soups and platters. There's also a tempting range of homemade cakes and puddings – hard to resist. For the purposes of the book however what made it stand out was its child-friendly policy. They were so lovely with the boys and the menu for children was very good with things like hummus and pitta dippers for £3 and beans and cheese toastie for £2.85. There was room for our pushchairs and there's a box for the children to dip into with colouring books, crayons and reading books. A good venue for lunch with babies or children.
Mon-Sat 10am-4pm
Hullabaloo, 5 Kings Court, Railway Street, Altrincham, Cheshire WA14 2RD Tel: 0161 941 4288

EATING OUT

Restaurants

babies in pushchairs so clearly I was not the first to test Loch Fyne as a child-friendly restaurant.

Our first stop was the colourful fish counter. My two boys were fascinated by the fresh lobsters, crabs, langoustines and oysters displayed although Sam looked a bit scared!

I was delighted to find they do a child's menu and for £6 you have a choice of haddock goujons, pan fried salmon or moules mariniere with chips plus an ice cream. Children's drinks aren't included in the price. If your child doesn't like fish, there are alternatives such as sausages or pasta.

Proudly Harry braved the mussels and loved them, even Sam tried a few with ketchup! Although Loch Fyne is one of the more expensive places on our list, they regularly carry offers that definitely make a meal more affordable.

Mon-Fri 9am-10pm, Sat 9am-10.30pm, Sun 10am-10pm
848 Wilmslow Road, Didsbury, Manchester M20 2RN
Tel: 0161 446 4190 www.lochfyne.com
Also at Alderley Edge, Knutsford and Warrington

The Olive Press

Part of chef Paul Heathcote's restaurant collection, the Olive Press chain is brilliantly child friendly. For a start and unlike anywhere else we've found (yet!!!), toddlers under three eat free (otherwise it's £7.50 for the three courses) and the menu selection they have to choose from is very impressive. The "make your own pizza" option is hugely popular in our household – a small pizza base is brought to your table with various toppings – the children then make their own concoction and it's whisked off to the oven. But if that doesn't take their fancy you've got plenty of pasta or grill dishes to choose from. They also get a drink (fruit juice, coke, milkshake) and dessert (knickerbocker glory, strawberries, chocolate cake) included. The standard of food is high both for adults and children and service has always been delightful.

Note: for pram pushers, there are a few steps up to the main door in the Manchester branch and then down again at the other end.

Mon-Thurs 11.45am-10pm, Fri-Sat 11.45am-11pm,
Sun 12noon-9pm
The Olive Press, 4 Lloyd Street, Off Deansgate,
Manchester M2 5AB
Tel: 0161 832 9090 www.olivepresspizzeria.co.uk
Also at Bolton, Cheadle Hulme, Clitheroe, Leeds,
Liverpool, Preston and Warrington.

Pizza Express

An ever-reliable favourite, Pizza Express is a pleasant dining experience and delivers consistently good pizzas. They are very family friendly and are more than used to the odd tantrum. You can

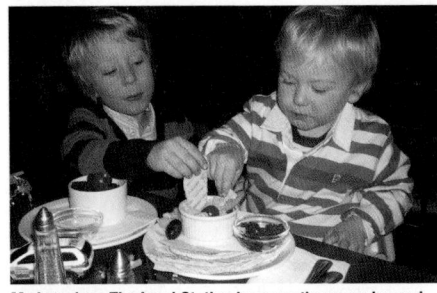
My boys love The Lead Station because the menu is good and the staff always take time to have a giggle with them. I love it because it is a night out in a trendy cafe bar.

watch pizzas being made in the open kitchen, but unfortunately you can't make your own (although some branches now cater for children's parties where you can do just that). The Piccolo children's meal is three courses for £5.65. This includes dough balls, pizza or pasta, salad and dessert, plus a Bambinoccino – frothy milk with chocolate sprinkles, that give parents an extra 10 minutes for a latte. With the usual supply of crayons and colouring paper, this is a good place to start if you're not used to going out for dinner with a toddler.

Mon-Sat 11.30am-11.30pm, Sun, 12noon-10.30pm
Pizza Express, South King Street, Manchester M2 6DQ
Tel: 0161 834 0145 www.pizzaexpress.com
Pizza Express restaurants are located all over Greater Manchester so check website for details

Pizza Hut

The older kids just love Pizza Hut. To begin with you're brought activity booklets and crayons, usually linked to a new movie release, so the kids are happy. The service is swift which is always appreciated. The food is unsophisticated, but good enough to keep eveybody happy. There are specific child menus, with a choice of larger or smaller portions from £3.49, offering pizza, chicken strips or pasta, with a salad bowl and drink. For £1 extra, kids usually choose to have something from the Ice Cream Factory. They are given a bowl and can get their own ice cream and sprinkles including mini marshmallows or chocolate raisins from a machine. At lunchtimes it's especially handy if you are in a hurry and have hungry youngsters as they offer a buffet for £3.49 – so you can be eating within a minute of walking in, and all done in 20 minutes! There's always a salad bar available though it's not very inspiring. The new pasta menu means that there is a better choice for alternatives to pizza.

Sun-Thurs 11.30am-8pm, Fri & Sat 11.30am-10pm
Pizza Hut Manchester, 79 Deansgate, Manchester
M3 2BW Tel: 0161 835 3035 www.pizzahut.co.uk
Pizza Hut restaurants are located all over Greater Manchester so check website for details

Queenie Mumbles

Probably one of my favourite cafes to go to with children. The fact that it's been ignored for any nomination in family friendly restaurant awards seems quite an oversight.

Managed by a mum of four, a lot of thought has gone into making this small, but perfectly formed café an enjoyable place to eat with children. The food on offer is mostly locally sourced and seasonal with everything being cooked to order. There is a very comprehensive menu but what's brilliant is that although there's an excellent platter (which rotates on a stand) and sandwich selection listed for the children, Queenie Mumbles will cook whatever they want: "if we have the ingredients we'll cook it."

There's a toy cart in one area of the café with lots of small activities designed for children to select something and take it back to their table to play with. Another excellent feature which allowed the mums to enjoy a coffee in peace was the 'decorate your own cupcake' option on the menu – for £1.95 the children are presented with a plain bun and icing, sugar strands, dolly mixtures and the like to embellish it with.

The most recent occasion we were at Queenie Mumbles, it was totally full and there were at least four prams squashed in with various new mums sitting around enjoying themselves and no-one minded one bit about squeezing past each other. Needless to say there are high chairs and baby changing is in the unisex toilet with wipes and nappy bags provided. In summer months, outside tables are available.

Mon 12noon-3pm, Tues-Sat 10am-6.30pm,
Sun 10am-5.30pm
Queenie Mumbles, 9 Goose Green, Altrincham
WA14 1DW
Tel: 0161 941 2215 www.queeniemumbles.co.uk

Shimla Pinks

It was a cold wet Sunday approaching tea time and we could only think of one thing that would warm the cockles of our heart – CURRY. We hoped our two year old would feel the same! We headed for Shimla Pinks. At an embarrassingly early 5.30pm we were first to arrive in the restaurant, but it filled up pretty quickly as Shimlas do a buffet on Sunday and Monday for £11 that really draws in the crowds. We ordered a la carte, which was a bit pricier. They don't have a dedicated kids' menu, but will do half portions of anything on the main menu, and if your children aren't familiar with spicy food, they will fry up some plain chicken with boiled rice. The staff were friendly, the food hit the spot, and we even got a balloon when we left. The only downside was that they don't have baby changing facilities, but they are

moving premises early in 2009 to Spinningfields, and the new place will be well kitted out for kids – the chef is even hoping they'll have a proper children's menu, so I'd say it will be worth a visit.

Mon-Fri 12noon-3pm and 5.30-11pm,
Weekends 5.30-11pm
Shimla Pinks, Crown Square, off Bridge Street,
Manchester M3 3HA
Tel: 0161 831 7099 www.shimlapinksmanchester.com

Tai Wu

The Tai Wu on Oxford Road opposite the Palace Theatre has been a favourite in our family since Harry was born nearly five years ago. We used to turn up on a weekend with him in his rock-a-tot and he would happily sit there while we gorged ourselves. This has now progressed into both our boys loving dim sum and we try and go regularly for Sunday lunch and usually meet up with the in-laws.

It's a brilliantly popular restaurant, full of Chinese families. We either arrive a few minutes before it opens at 12, though we are still never first in line! Or leave it until later when things have quietened down. You will probably still have to take a ticket and wait in the bar area for 15 minutes.

Tai Wu serves traditional dim sum from trolleys pushed around the restaurant. Obviously they are hot, so be careful with toddlers. The benefit is food available immediately, but you can still order from the menu if there's a dish you prefer. With all the various dishes arriving in different bamboo baskets, children are interested and might try stuff they probably wouldn't at home. The service is quick, they have plenty of highchairs and really seem to like children. They don't provide colouring pens or activity packs so take some toys. The toilets are downstairs but there is a baby changing table in the disabled toilet at the end of the bar.

Also downstairs is an all you can eat buffet which is available pretty much all the time, good if you're in a hurry or want to try a variety of different dishes, it does have a one and a half hour time limit so you can't stay all day!

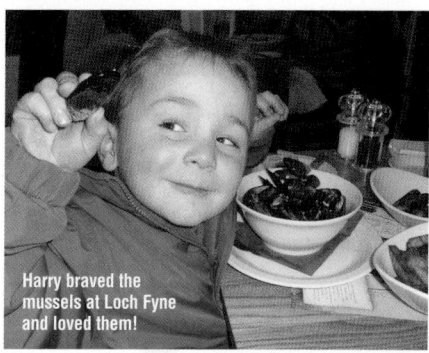

Harry braved the mussels at Loch Fyne and loved them!

Restaurants

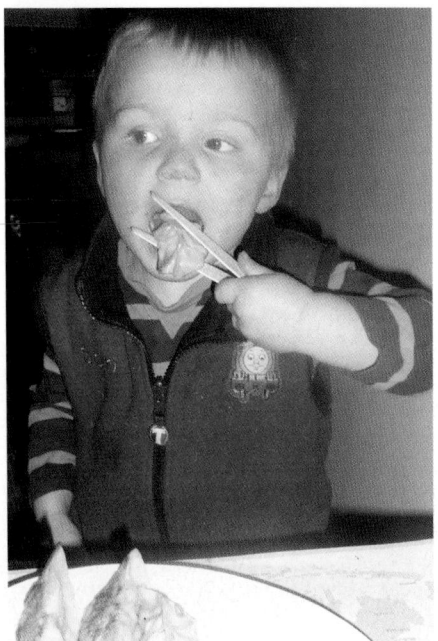

A trip to Tampopo is great with children.

Mon-Sun 12noon-2.45am, Dim Sum Mon-Sun 12noon-6pm, (12noon-4pm Dim Sum is half price)
Tai Wu, 44 Oxford Road, Mancheste, M1 5EJ
Tel: 0161 236 6557 www.tai-wu.co.uk

Tampopo

This noodle restaurant is a regular venue for my two boys and me. You can be in and out within half an hour and the food and service is excellent. I think home grown Tampopo is a deserving winner of last years Best Family Friendly Venue at the Manchester Food and Drink Festival. It always feels a bit of treat as I love noodles and with a children's menu at £3.95 available there is no problem with us all going en famille. It includes a dessert of either rich chocolate ice cream or mango sorbet. If chicken noodles don't appeal, the kitchen can make any of the main courses in smaller portions for £4.50. Colouring pens and paper are brought to the table and special chopsticks make eating a fun and messy treat. There are now three venues in Manchester and all are superb. The original Albert Square branch is the least child friendly with steep steps into the basement and no baby changing facilities.

Between 12noon-7pm everyday, there is an Eastern Express adult menu at £6.95 for two courses. See page 95 for our voucher offering a free child's meal at Tampopo.

Mon-Sat 12noon-11pm, Sun 12noon-10pm
Tampopo, Triangle Shopping Centre, 38 Exchange Square, Manchester M4 3TR
Tel: 0161 839 6484 www.tampopo.co.uk
Also at Albert Square and The Trafford Centre

TGI Friday's

TGI's is a great place to take the kids and they are very child friendly. There are high chairs aplenty and it's always nice to be greeted with colouring sheets and crayons. Portion sizes are huge, however there is a children's menu which not only offers pasta and burgers, but for the more adventurous, fajitas and quesadillas. Mains for children start at £2.99 with desserts from 99p and drinks from £1.29. For the babies TGI's offer free Hipp Organic food for 4-10 month olds if an adult is dining. As the atmosphere is loud and noisy it did not seem to matter that my little one was screaming lustily when we got there, but was soon pacified by the balloons and general vibrancy of this fun eatery.
Daily 11.30am-11pm
TGI Fridays, Valley Park Road off, Bury New Road, Prestwich M25 3AJ
Tel: 0161 798 7125 www.tgifridays.co.uk
Also at Cheadle, Sale and The Trafford Centre

Wagamama

With a name that translates to mean wilful or naughty child, surely Wagamama must be the place to go with children for dinner.

The original branch in Manchester is in Exchange Square and the restaurant is below ground. The doors are automatic and there is lift access; the baby changing and toilets are on the first level with the restaurant on the lower level. The staff are always friendly and the food is consistently good. Highchairs clip straight onto the table so there's no problem sitting wherever you like, a noodle doodle colouring sheet and crayons are brought to your table.

A recent addition to the Wagamama chain can be found in the newly developed Spinningfields area of the city. This branch is on one level and baby changing is in the disabled toilets – it's very popular with families at the weekend.

A child's main course starts from £3.40 for a mini chicken ramen – chicken breast served on a noodle soup. Priced separately, desserts include vanilla ice cream, £1.05 or natural flavoured lollies at £1.55. Drinks are either freshly squeezed orange or apple juice at £1.45. With a speedy service and no additives, even for my wilful child, Wagamama is a great place to eat.
Mon-Sat 12noon-11pm Sun 12noon-10pm
Wagamama, 1 The Printworks, Corporation Street, Manchester M4 2BS
Tel: 0161 839 5916 www.wagamama.com
Also at Spinningfields, Manchester

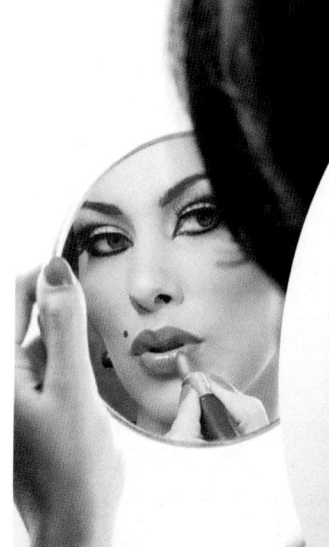
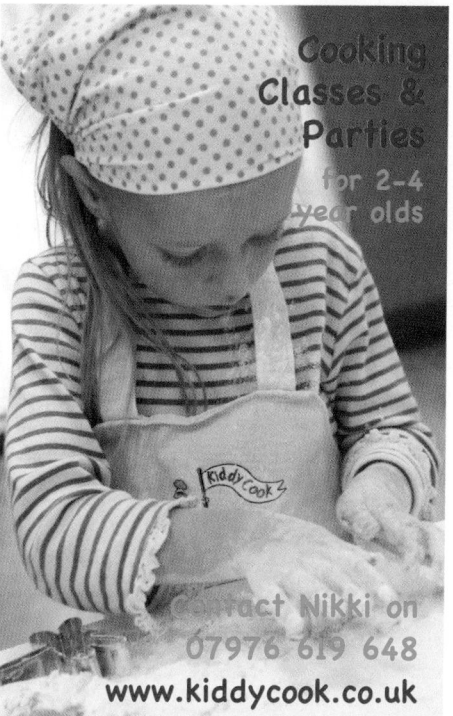
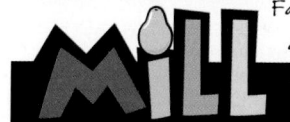
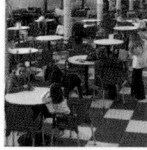
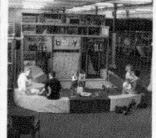
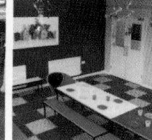

Cafés

If you're in need of a reviving cuppa, a bite to eat or maybe something stronger... here's our Top 10 favourite cafes to wheel your buggy in to.

Cafés in town

St Ann's Saturday Cafe

At the geographic centre of Manchester, the café of St Ann's Church is a peaceful retreat from frenetic shoppers on a Saturday, which I find great if my boys are getting tetchy. If you go into the main church entrance, the small cafe, which is staffed by volunteers from the congregation, is situated at the back of the church. It sells homemade sandwiches and slices of cake all served with a smile and at a nice price. The tea and coffee is all accredited by Fair Trade. If you find the cafe's full, the Reverend is happy for you to sit in the pews! There is a bookstall selling some children's books. There is a high chair but currently no baby changing.
Saturday 10am-3.30pm.
St Ann's Church, St. Ann St, Manchester www.stannsmanchester.com

CUP

Appealing, independent café – no homogenised global branding here. It's all good home cooking and great smoothies. Admittedly it's not super-dooper child friendly – the beautiful display of porcelain cups for sale on a table in the centre of the café may cause anxiety to those with hyper-active toddlers (we sat the furthest point away!) – but it's buggy friendly, there are high chairs if you want a restraint-mechanism and the staff are good-natured. Cup's pretty sizeable so you'll have no problem parking prams next to the tables though when we went at the weekend it did start getting very busy after 1pm, so bear that in mind. Food-wise, you can grab a pieminister pie for £4, scrambled eggs on a bagel for £3 and sweet crepes for £3.25 amongst other things. There is only one unisex toilet in the café but it does have a baby-change table.
Mon 8am-5pm, Tues-Fri 8am-7pm, Weekends 9am-7pm
CUP Cafe, 53-55 Thomas Street, Northern Quarter,
Manchester M4 1NA Tel: 0161 832 3233

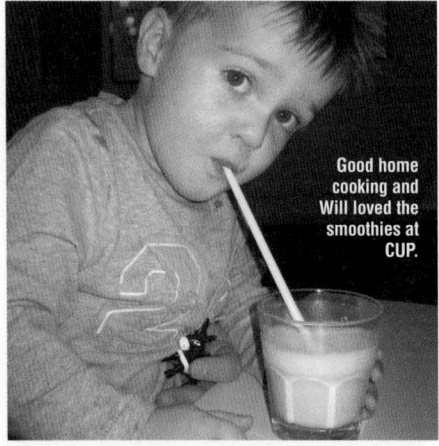

Good home cooking and Will loved the smoothies at CUP.

Oklahoma

Is a bit bonkers and all the better for it! On one side there is a shop with shelves crammed full of quirky retro stuff, jokey and wacky gifts, imported goods and a great selection of cards and on the other side there's a mainly veggie café with an eclectic mix of comfy chairs and tables. It's bustling at weekends and yes you'd struggle a little with a pram when it's very busy but Oklahoma is something different. They absolutely welcome children and it's really worth a trip if you're after an alternative present combined with a good coffee or yummy milkshake. Foodwise options include a sweet potato & cheese for £4.90, scrambled egg on toast £3.10 and cheese toastie £3.50. Two entrances, both involving small steps. There are two highchairs and one unisex toilet with a baby changing surface in it.
Mon-Sat 8am-7pm, Sun 10am-6pm
Oklahoma, 74-76 High Street, Manchester M4 1ES
Tel: 0161 834 1136 www.oklahomacafe.co.uk

Selfridges Exchange Moet Bar and Restaurant

This is the restaurant located on the second floor – rather temptingly, the same level as the womens' clothing. We've been a few times for lunch as we love the views out of the big glass windows towards the Manchester Wheel. We always have a very pleasant time here as the staff are extremely good with babies and children. The system changed slightly on my last visit as there's no longer a dedicated children's menu – you can now choose off the main menu and they'll make it a kid's size and halve the price (approximately) or they can rustle up what they call a "plain menu" where basically they'll endeavour to cook whatever simple food you'd like to request for the children such as sausage & mash, chicken & chips. Toilets with baby change are close by on the second floor.
Mon-Fri 10am-5.30pm, Sat 9am-5.30pm, Sun 12noon-4pm
Selfridges Manchester, Exchange Square, 1 Exchange Square,
Manchester M3 1BD Tel: 0161 838 0540 www.selfridges.com

House of Fraser (Kendals) – Restaurant on the 6th Floor

I'm fond of shopping at Manchester's landmark department store, so being able to combine it with a coffee or snack with my little boy is an added pleasure. The restaurant is extremely child-friendly with the staff giving me tap water with a straw for Will and offering to carry my tray to the table. It's all one level with a fair amount of space for prams too. They have children's lunch boxes or a hot meal for £3.50 including an activity pack. You can also buy the items separately which is useful. There are high chairs and they will heat up bottles etc. For really little ones, they stock the Baby Deli range of meals. Baby changing (together with Hamleys toyshop and childrenswear) is on the same floor. There are however a few steps up to the toilets, but if that's going to be tricky, try the additional baby-changing on the third floor which doesn't have this problem.
Mon-Fri 9.30am-7pm, Sat 9am-7pm , Sun 11am-5pm
House of Fraser, Deansgate, Manchester M60 3AU
Tel: 0161 832 3414 www.houseoffraser.co.uk

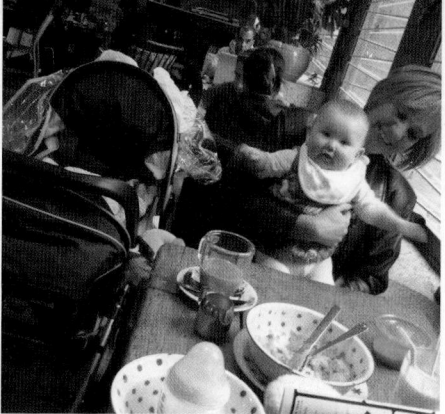

Oklahoma is bustling at weekends and you may struggle a little with a pram when it's busy but it is something different and they absolutely welcome children.

Manchester Cathedral Visitor Centre

Hidden in the basement of the centre is a pleasant self-service cafe/restaurant which is very handy for The Arndale, Selfridges and The Triangle. There is a friendly atmosphere and the staff are more than happy to help you if you have children in tow. If you want a hearty lunch at a good price, there is plenty on offer such as braised lamb shanks, three cheese red onion tartlet. Or if you prefer, simpler options like jacket potatoes, sandwiches and pastries. Because it is self-serve there isn't a long wait at the table for your food. This always seems to be of utmost importance to my hungry boys. The cafe shares the same space as the Hanging Bridge; a 15th century medieval bridge that originally connected the Church with the medieval town. It is one of Manchester oldest structures, and a scheduled monument. There is a lift to the basement. Baby change and high chairs available.
Open from 10.30am daily and serves food from 12.15-3.30pm
Manchester Cathedral Visitor Centre, 10 Cateaton Street,
Manchester M3 1SQ Tel: 0161 835 4030 www.mcvc.info

The Midland Hotel

For a special treat, dress your little cherubs in their Sunday best and head for afternoon tea at the grand old Midland Hotel. Served daily, from 2.30-5pm, children will love the dainty finger sandwiches and delightful cakes served on pretty cake tiers. We shared an adult's tea between us and it was plenty for an adult and two children. It is advisable to book ahead. Baby change facilities and high chairs.
Daily 2.30-5pm. Costs £16.95 per tea and upwards
The Midland Hotel, 16 Peter St, Manchester M60 2DS
Tel: 0161 236 3333

Café Revive at Marks and Spencer

When I'd just had my first baby and I was out shopping in the city centre, Café Revive became a regular haunt. I made sure I timed it early enough to get a seat before the lunchtime rush and I enjoyed sitting there with a coffee and sandwich looking out of the floor-to-ceiling glass windows towards St. Ann's Square. The staff were unerringly helpful – always offering to carry my tray to the table as I negotiated my pram. They'll provide bottle warmers and there's baby changing in the toilets within the café.

Store open Mon-Thurs 9am-8pm, Fri-Sat 8.30am-8pm,
Sun 11am-5pm
Café Revive at Marks and Spencer, 7 Market Street, Manchester
M1 1WT Tel: 0161 831 7341 www.marksandspencer.com

Cafe at the Rylands

Situated in the modern extension of one of Manchester's most beautiful gothic buildings, the cafe is spacious and light with a floor that lets prams just glide over. Often quiet and with a children's menu offering items such as Lancashire cheese on toast or Manchester sausage on toast together with a piece of fruit or juice and a cookie for £3.25 it is a good option. If you haven't before and you have time, I would recommend taking a peek at the Library itself following your visit to the cafe. There is a lift to all floors. Baby change facilities and high chairs.
Mon, Weds-Sat 10am-4.30pm, Tues, Sun 12noon-4.30pm
John Rylands Library, 150 Deansgate M3 3EH

Podium Restaurant Bar and Lounge

Situated on the ground floor of the imposing Hilton Hotel, Podium is open in the mornings for a full English or simply pastries with a smoothie and coffee. It is great if you are with a pram because it is so spacious and there are conveniently positioned baby change facilities. You can either eat in the lounge area or the more formal restaurant area. We opted for a pastry in the lounge and my children enjoyed looking out of the floor to ceiling windows at the hustle and bustle of Deansgate. It is very handy for the Museum of Science and Industry (see page 7) which is only a five minute walk away.
Open for breakfast: Mon-Fri 6.30-10.30am, Weekends 7-11am
Also open for lunch and dinner.
Hilton Manchester Deansgate, 303 Deansgate Manchester M3 4LQ
Tel: 0161 870 1600 www.hilton.co.uk/manchesterdeansgate

The Social Café at Urbis

Manchester's exhibition centre about city life has a very friendly café. Porridge is served for breakfast with banana or maple syrup. From 11am onwards, children's choices are mini burger, fish and chips, pappardelle all for £3.50 each or Cumberland sausage and mash for £4. In the afternoons they serve very tasty cakes, scones and iced buns. The selection of adult food and drink is also excellent.

Staff are friendly and eager to help. They'll willingly mash up any food for baby and will of course heat a bottle for you. Quite often the exhibitions spill over in to the café which is a lot of fun. When we went it was about the history of fashion. People in 1940's clothing wandered through and the tables were decorated with ostrich feathers. There was a DJ in the corner playing vinyl copies of everything from Mama Cass to Billie Holliday.

Toilets are large and clean and include a separate baby changing room all adjacent to the café on the ground floor. Urbis itself has a frequent programme of events for children. Check the website for details. For 2009, they're launching Baby Boom every Tuesday morning between 10 and 12. It's billed as a free "baby friendly social club."
Mon-Sun 10am-6pm
The Social Café at Urbis, Cathedral Gardens, Manchester M4 3BG
Tel: 0161 605 8200 www.urbis.org.uk

Classes

You've had your baby, they're six months old and suddenly not content to sit in the pushchair while you amble round the shops, help, what's next…

Singing, sticking and sports

This is definitely the time to start looking around at the many classes on offer. Mums generally run them so they understand exactly what you're going through. Although they all offer a variety of things, essentially they have similar benefits, from learning to share and taking turns, building confidence and self-esteem, or for you to simply spend time with your child and bond. It's also a good way to get out of the house and meet other parents with children of a similar age.

Whatever you choose to do, most have a free trial session and it is definitely worth trying out different ones. Although our list is by no means exhaustive, it does cover a range of activities and classes, so something should catch your eye.

ART AND CRAFT

Mini Masters These fun and informal art and craft sessions are run in Didsbury by Petra, an experienced craft designer. They are small groups, aimed at pre-school children, that take place during school hours on a bi-weekly basis. Each week a different masterpiece or technique/medium is introduced through stories and demonstration. The children then use this as inspiration to create their own artwork – everything from clay modelling right though to making prints from household objects.

Sessions cost £4.50 each and include all materials and refreshments (for children and adults).
Tel: 0161 286 8898

Mucky Pups If you have a child that likes to help decorate your home unasked, then you will enjoy Mucky Pups. Each week there is a different topic like Creepy Crawlies and all the activities follow that theme. Seven stations are set up with an activity on each table, plus playdough. There is enough gluing, sticking and painting to keep active hands occupied for hours, plus you don't have to clear up afterwards. At the end of the class there is an opportunity to show off your best piece.

Classes are approximately an hour and include a drink and a biscuit. They cost £5, except for Timperley, which costs £6 because it also includes entry into the Antz in your Pantz soft play centre (see page 69).
Bramhall, Brooklands, Wilmslow, Timperley and Knutsford Tel: 07511 622445 www.mucky-pups.com

COOKING

Kiddy Cook This is a cooking class designed for children aged 2-11 years to encourage them to learn about food and to explore new flavours in an educational and fun way. I tried the 'Cookie Tots' sessions for the 2-4 year old range and found it incredible to see how much teacher Nikki fitted into 45 minutes.

Sessions start with a warm-up to music using actions that mirror culinary activities such as rolling out pastry or kneading bread. Then a puppet called Katie Custard is brought out to tell the children what they'll be cooking and hand out recipe cards – the children have to identify the ingredients they will need from Nikki's bag. The day I went we made 'Mice in Jackets' – cheese filled jacket potatoes. Afterwards there's a short story, then a bit of hands-on craft work. Next the children take part in a 'show and taste' session, when Nikki brings out a piece of exotic fruit for the children to examine and try. A song then rounds it all off.

Cookie Tots costs £5.95 a session (ingredients and utensils provided) and you sign up per half-term. There is a £10 joining fee, for which you get an apron, recipe cards and a personalised recipe card holder.
Bowdon, Bramhall and Wilmslow
Tel: 07976 619648 (Nikki) www.kiddycook.co.uk

MUSIC AND ENTERTAINMENT

Jabberjacks Jabberjacks is a music based activity class for babies to pre-school children. Each session starts with a welcome song and shaking hands with the leader. The focus then shifts to the mystery box, singing 'What is in the box today?' Goodies vary from puppets and wands to bubbles and instruments. The box is opened two to three times each session with a new and exciting discovery every time. There is a sharing toy which is passed round then each child gets to explore a bag full of things

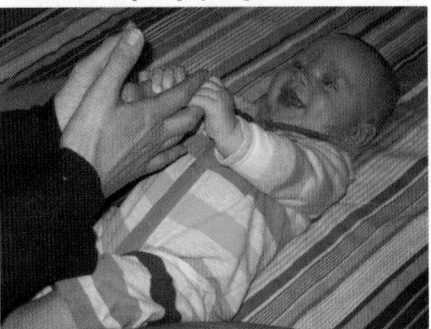

Daniel telling mummy he's happy at Tiny Talk.

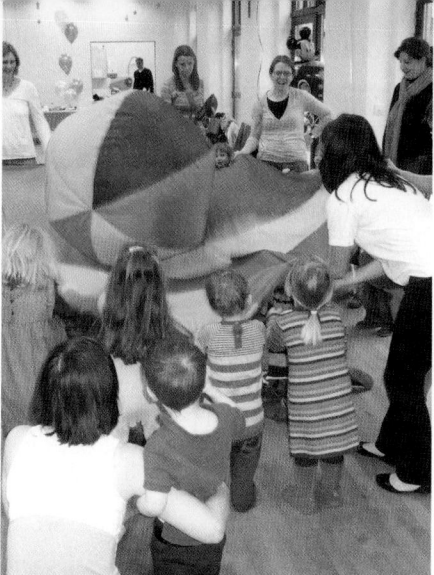

A Kiddiewinks class does not stop from the moment you arrive until you sing the final song.

like a teddy bear's picnic, pet grooming kit or musical instruments.

Fees range from £4.75-£5.20 and are paid termly in advance with a one-off £10 registration fee which includes a Jabberjacks T-shirt.
Bramhall, Bowden, Cheadle, Didsbury, Marple, Poynton, Prestbury, Prestwich, Sale and Wilmslow
Tel: 0161 442 9911 www.jabberjacks.co.uk

Kiddiewinks This is a class that does not stop from the moment you arrive until you sing the final song, every five minutes a new activity begins. There is no time to stop and think, let alone get bored. Each week has a different theme that also incorporates the pre-school curriculum.

The class I went to was titled 'Growing'. First we started with animal puppets and what their young were called; then we talked about healthy eating and exercise which then moved into a 'growing up dance' with pom-poms! A bit of quiet time was next as out came little bags containing babies with baths, bottles and clothes. I couldn't believe how much my boys enjoyed feeding and dressing the baby. Sticking with the growing theme, they also had a go at planting pansies in a pot and decorating it with loads of stickers, plus they got to take them home.

Classes are one hour long (from walking to pre-school age) during term time and are £4 per session payable per term. This includes juice and biscuits at the end and a chance to take home 'Rascal', the Kiddiewinks bear, for the week.
Didsbury, Chorlton, Stockport, Cheadle, Wilmslow, Handforth and Worsley. Check website for new classes.
Tel: 0161 432 3624 www.kiddiewinksonline.com

Rhythm and Rhyme This was the first class that I enrolled in with my baby and we loved it. Children and parents sit in a circle for the 45-minute sessions which involve singing, instruments, banging on the big drum, playing with a large 'parachute' sheet, dancing to jazz, classical or pop music and at the end, everyone's favourite – blowing bubbles. Our teacher was lovely and really enthusiastic. The sessions are designed for babies from five months to pre-school and cost £48 per 12-week term.
Bramhall, Cheadle, Chorlton, Didsbury, Heaton Moor, Sale, Timperley, Urmston
Tel: 0161 860 0911 www.rhythmandrhyme.co.uk

Rhythm Time The half-hour Rhythm Time class has sessions for babies and toddlers up to age three. The baby session starts with a welcome song, after which the leader encourages singing and interaction with the babies together with lots of bouncing to keep them entertained. There are lots of other baby-specific activities, including one called 'baby in a basket', where parents and carers are encouraged to lay their babies in a washing basket and spin them round gently on the ground while everyone else continues to sing. Apparently this helps with spatial awareness but I must say I'm not convinced!

The toddlers session is geared towards children from 15 months to three years. It is designed to encourage children to sing on their own and by playing instruments with parents, helps them follow the rhythm. Both sessions cost £3.75 per child paid termly.
Greater Manchester
Tel: Head office on 0121 711 4244
www.rhythmtime.net

Sally Jolley Music Group This is a fantastic little group although I am totally biased as I have been going to it for over two years. Friends from a toddler class introduced me and the arrangement is that Sally comes to your house and takes an interactive music session lasting 45 minutes for a small group aged from two and a half years to school age.

The group runs every other week, so it's not a huge commitment on your time and the cost is divided by how many children there are for the term. The variety of instruments and puppets Sally has built up over the years is amazing. The children love it.

Eight children is an ideal number as you take it in turns to host the group, so once a term you have to give your house a spring clean (only for it to be trashed two hours later!) So get a bunch of friends together and give it a go. She reckons our group has been going for the best part of 12 years!
Classes available to book, cost is £38 per session divided by the number in your group.
Tel: 01663 765877

CLASSES AND ACTIVITIES

Classes

Tiny Talk The concept behind Tiny Talk is that the classes teach baby sign language. To the uninitiated, like myself, the class appeared to be fundamentally made up of singing with the usual actions attached. So when I went we had Insy Winsy Spider, Head Shoulders Knees and Toes and Old MacDonald amongst others. We learnt a couple of specific signs in the class but not as much as I was expecting, which was absolutely fine – it was a good fun group, led by a great teacher and the babies enjoyed the songs.

Tiny Talk classes last for one hour with the final half-hour being given over to 'social and support' time – basically a friendly natter with everyone over tea and biscuits with toys out for the babies. Tiny Talk is aimed at birth to two year olds, classes are approximately £4.50 each and you can either drop in or book a term of six for £24.

Swinton, Worsley, Walkden, Warrington, Altrincham, Stretford, Wigan, Bramhall and Wilmslow.
Tel: 07769 712 577 www.tinytalk.co.uk

NATURE AND WILDLIFE

Forest School Set in a small woodland hidden in the heart of suburban Manchester, the Forest School provides a structured woodland playgroup.

Run by a qualified Forest Teacher, each weekly session introduces the children to a different aspect of woodland life through stories and exploration. The sessions run all year, allowing children to experience nature through the seasons.

Whilst there is naturally no formal toilet facilities, there is a 'wee-tree' and plenty of space to change nappies! There are healthy drinks and snacks provided. Classes are weekly, Wednesday from 1-2.30pm (during term time) and held in Paupers Wood, Nell Lane, Didsbury.

It costs £24 for a six-week course. Numbers are limited for safety reasons. Suitable from 18 months to pre-school.
Tel: Mary Maclachlan 0161 445 3520
www.foresteducation.org

SPORTS

Baby Yoga This is a great low impact workout for you and your baby. Sessions start with some light stretches and a dry massage for the babies followed by gentle movement to songs and an easy workout for the adults. I loved the lie down at the end, which if you can get your child to lie still will have you asleep in less than five minutes.

For the babies the advantages are clear – it is good for digestion, co-ordination and movement. For the adults, an hour out of the house doing something a bit different and really bonding with your baby.

Classes start from eight weeks old after babies have had their hip check and go on until about a year. A new group called Toddler Yoga, which is aimed at one to four year olds, will be up and running in early 2009.

Classes are approximately an hour, with a maximum of 10 adults, and cost £40 for five weeks in Didsbury and £32.50 for five weeks in Chorlton.
Tel: 07956 216218

Kindergym When children arrive at the South Manchester Gymnastics Centre, they can't wait to get started. Set in a huge industrial unit, there are two large rooms full of equipment. In the first, an obstacle course is set up that children can get straight on and work their way round. When the class gets started it's with a warm up involving hoops and music which then leads back onto the obstacle course ending with roly-polys.

You can then move into the second room where there's a huge trampoline, swing ropes, bars and rings, all over giant pits of soft foam. You're free to jump in too, although you do look a bit foolish trying to get back out again.

You take turns on the trampoline and it's free play until the class ends with the hokey-cokey. All the children love it and woe betide if you try and leave early! Sessions last for one hour and parent

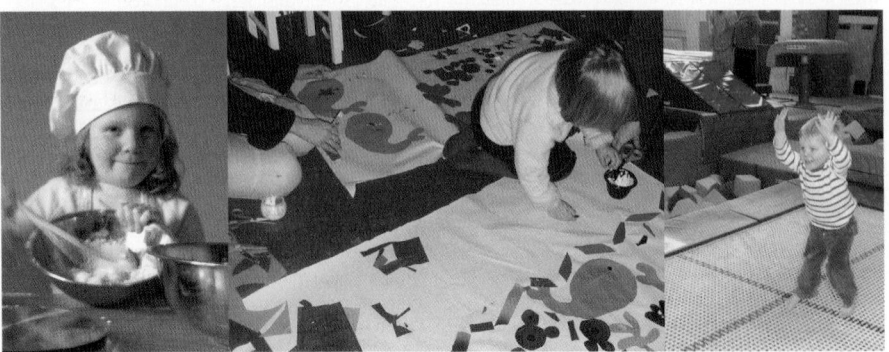

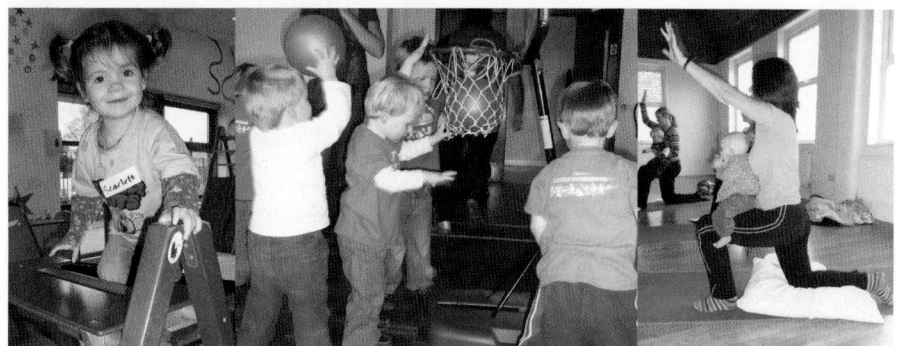

participation is necessary. Kindergym is aimed at children from 18 months to four years old and costs £30 for an eight-week course. There is also an annual insurance payment of £10.
South Manchester Gymnastics Centre, Fenside Road, Wythenshawe, Manchester M22 4PD
Tel: 0161 491 0415 www.southmanchestergymnastics.org

Little Kickers This is all about one thing – football! Two pop-up nets are set up and loads of balls are kicked around, and that's before the class even starts. I'm not sure who enjoys it more, the children or the parents. Two coaches are on hand so parent involvement can be as much or as little as you prefer.

The class starts with all the children on the mats doing a gentle warm-up. Then there are a series of games such as 'traffic lights', which shows who has been listening when the red marker is held up. Lastly, and clearly the favourite bit – penalties – a chance to score a goal with loads of cheering and support from mums and dads.

There are two different 45-minute classes available: Junior Kickers for two to three and a half year olds, and Mighty Kickers for three and a half to five year olds. Both cost £6.50 per session and are paid every half-term. There is also a £16 one-off membership fee which includes a pretty cool football strip.
Didsbury, Altrincham, Sale, Bowden, Lymm, Prestwich and Whitefield
Tel: 0161 442 5713 www.littlekickers.co.uk

Little Superstars is an activity class covering general sports including rugby, golf, cricket and football. After a good warm-up, various games are played that change every 10 minutes and have an educational theme, with an emphasis on colours and counting.

Each session then focuses on one main sport and involves parents in one-to-one with their children after a demo from the coach. For example, the basketball session involves bouncing and catching the ball, then scoring baskets in smaller, specially adapted nets.

This is not the sort of thing you go to and put your feet up while your children run around – parental participation is essential.

Little Superstars holds 30-minute sessions for walking to two year olds and 50-minute sessions for two to five year olds. The cost is £4.75 per class payable per term and includes a free T-shirt.
Bowdon, Altrincham, Knutsford, Hale Barns, Appleton, Wilmslow, Marple, Middleton, Prestwich, Oldham, Hyde and Prestbury
Tel: 07904 311552 www.littlesuperstars.co.uk

Mini Movers These open play sessions are run by Stockport Council's Play Development team. The hour-long classes involve parent and child interaction with either soft play, bat and ball or various climbing frames. They end in circle time with group singing and activities. There is a progressive badge scheme and each term badges are awarded by Max the Rabbit for skills demonstrated each week.

Mini Movers is for children aged 18 months to starting school. It's £3 per session and you sign up for a term.
Bramhall, Cale Green, Cheadle, Edgeley, Marple, Reddish
Tel: 0161 474 4471 www.play.dev@stockport.gov.uk

Tumble Tots This group is split into three age brackets – Gymbabes is for the youngest set, and is ideal if your six-month-old is desperate to get moving. The group starts with some warm-up songs and actions, then it is free style around the equipment before more songs and stickers at the end. As your child grows and starts to walk, the classes adapt accordingly. First to Tumble Tots, which encourages balance, climbing, co-ordination and independence. Then on to Gymbobs for school age children.

There is a member of staff per six children so there is a lot of encouragement and the group is friendly and welcoming. Classes last approximately 40 minutes and cost £5.50 each, paid in half-term blocks. There is also a £20 annual membership fee to cover insurance.
Lymm, Chorlton, Knutsford, Hale, Sale and Didsbury
Tel: 0161 499 3699 www.tumbletots.com

Classes

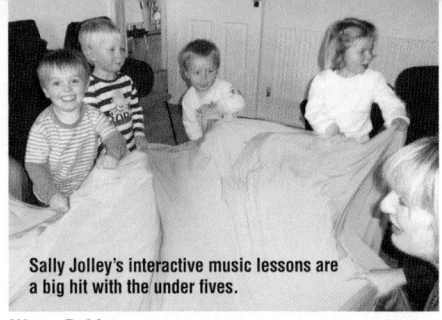

SWIMMING LESSONS

Aqua Babies run classes at small, warm pools. Each baby enters the water with a parent or carer and there are between six and 10 children in each class, depending on pool size. The classes are very well-run – they involve water play, submersions and singing and last around 20 minutes. Course fees are £10.50 per lesson and there is a waiting list.
Classes held in Bowden, Bramhall, Cheadle, Didsbury, Oldham and Timperley
Tel: 0161 973 1931 www.aquababies.co.uk

Puddle Ducks When I went to a Puddle Ducks class in Warrington I'd forgotten how great it was to have lessons. The instructor is in the pool with you and you're taught tricks and techniques to encourage your child to be more confident in the water. The teachers are brilliant, and their confidence definitely rubs off! Lessons include lots of songs and games, and the only flotation used is a woggle (a long float tube).

There are different classes dependent on age (from under six months right up to five years) and they cost from £9.25 per session for a 12-week course. There are no more than nine children per class.
Warrington and Cheshire
Tel: 01477 535527 www.puddleducks-swimming.co.uk

Sally Jolley's interactive music lessons are a big hit with the under fives.

Water Babies While the main emphasis is on having fun, a Water Babies course is highly structured. About 95 per cent of the lesson takes place on the surface, the rest underwater, but the swims beneath the surface only last a few seconds and the babies I watched going under the water were absolutely at ease with it.

The lessons are run by very experienced teachers whose enthusiasm is contagious. Classes include lots of splashing and kicking, as well as singing, work with floats and toys, and for the older ones, jumping in off the sides.

All told Water Babies was very impressive and I'll definitely be signing up for a course when my baby arrives. Each lesson costs between £10.50 and £13 charged as complete terms of nine, 10 or 13 weeks.
Blackley, Bolton, Bury, Manchester, Standish and Wigan
Tel: 01204 846 003   www.waterbabies.co.uk

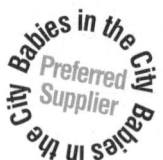
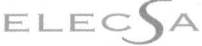
CLASSES AND ACTIVITIES

In our activities section, we've tried to list things that are available as a drop-in with no pre-booking necessary. You don't always want every day to be planned to the last detail and you might just want to go swimming or take a trip to the library. Here are a few ideas of what you can do.

Rainy day activities

INDOOR PLAY CENTRES

Antz in your Pantz There are three zones here – a little area for the under ones where they can crawl and climb in a padded area with toys; a slightly larger section built on two levels with slides aimed at the 1-5year olds (though ours got bored quite quickly here and moved onto the big boys bit!) and then the main area with all the usual equipment – astro slide, rope bridges, tunnels etc. A nice touch is the fairly plentiful supply of ride-along cars and tractors as well as the popular small football area. A good selection of food and drink is available.
Mon, Weds and Thurs 9.30am-6pm, Tues 9.30am-4pm and Fri-Sun 9.30am-6.30pm.
Over 3s £4.85, Under 3s £3.85, Active babies £1.
'Play and meal' deals on offer.
Unit 8 Crown Industrial Estate, Canal Road, Timperley, Cheshire WA14 1TD
Tel: 0161 962 2266 www.antzinyourpantz.co.uk

Cheeky Chimps Activity Centre is surprisingly homely for a soft play centre. It isn't enormous but the space is excellently used with a three-tier main play area containing toddler and baby sections. There is a superb supply of toys for the children to play with, and a few fast and steep slides. The staff are friendly and keep everywhere immaculate – the baby change facility with pretty pictures, a mobile above the changing mat and free nappy sacks was one of the best I've seen. The café's menu is simple, tasty and reasonably priced. The children opted for the lunchboxes, which included a sandwich, crisps, fruit juice, fruit or biscuit, a balloon, crayons and colouring picture all for only £2.99.
Daily from 10am (check if you're intending to arrive after 3pm as it is sometimes booked for private parties).
Weekdays term time Over 1s £2.50, Under 1s £2
Weekends, school holidays and bank holidays Over 3s £3.50.
Acorn Street, Lees, Oldham OL4 3PD
Tel: 0161 626 2552
www.cheekychimpsplaycentre.co.uk

Curly Whirleez is laid out on multiple levels with great facilities in its three sections. There's a toddler soft play area, tube slide, wavy astro slide, ball pool and car track plus a lovely (scaled down!) red double decker bus for the children to play in. There are

also various activities on offer, including toddler yoga, pre-school gymnastics and parent and toddler meetings. A decent café serves sandwiches, soup, drinks, fruit etc all at reasonable prices.
Mon-Fri 9.30am-6pm, Weekends 9.30am-5.30pm.
Over 3s £4, Under 3s £3.50, Under 1s free
Weekends Under 3s £4 Over 3s £4.50.
Boundary Industrial Estate, Millfield Road, Bolton BL2 6QY
Tel: 01204 523620 www.curlywhirleez.com

Geronimo is set out over two levels, with seating sections ideally placed near to the play area. The equipment includes a football pitch and sports area, two-level adventure play frame, quad slide, slide swing, ball pools, toddler cars and a baby and toddler area. The food at Geronimos is lovely, whether you are after a homemade lunch (including menus for children) or simply a slice of cake.

Also worth looking out for are the 'mums n tots' sessions held daily on weekdays (during term times).
Mon-Sat 9.30am-6pm, Sun 10am-6pm.
Over 1s £3.50, Under 1s £1, Under six months free.
Holidays, weekends and after 3pm Over 1s £4.
348 Wilderspool Causeway, Warrington, Cheshire WA4 6QP Tel: 01925 244855 www.gogeronimo.co.uk

Funizuz is split between two rooms. The first room has two ball pits and a two-lane astro slide for older children as well as two separate areas for under 18 months and under threes – seating is limited in this room. In the second room there is a small under fours' area with a slide and perspex tunnel plus a

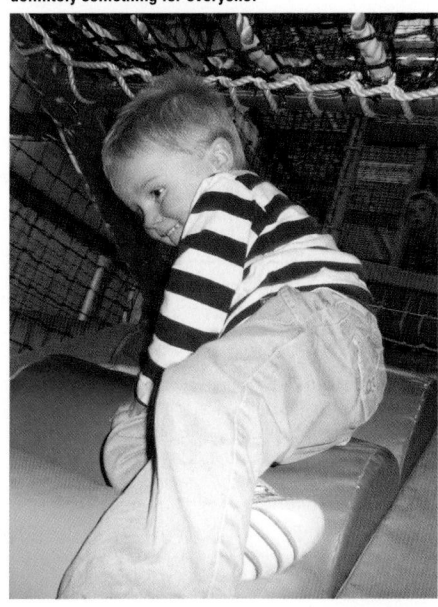

Manchester has some great indoor play centres. There is definitely something for everyone.

Activities

café with lots of seating and a television. Children's meals include pasta, chicken nuggets, sausages or fish fingers, chips, yoghurt and squash for £4. There is also a good pottery workshop.
Mon-Sun 10am-6pm. Over 3s £4.50, 9 months-3 years £3.50. Pre-school sessions 10am-2pm term time only £3 including juice and biscuits.
Brookfield Road Industrial Estate, Cheadle, Stockport SK8 2PN
Tel: 0161 491 6611 www.funizuz.co.uk.

Head Over Heels is one of the largest play centres in the UK and the proud owner of an award-winning restaurant *(The Observer 2006/7).*

There are leather sofas and comfy chairs next to the main play area which, at three storeys high with a three-lane astro slide, keeps the children suitably busy. Worth a special mention is the exclusively under threes soft play section – it's quite sizeable and really well equipped, with things like a ball pool with air fountain, slide, perspex tunnel, soft play roundabout and animals, play house, ride-on cars and play panels among other things.

The kids' menu serves favourites such as lasagne, chicken goujons and scrambled eggs on toast. The adults' menu has an excellent choice too. Staff are happy to heat up baby food or bottles on request.
Mon-Fri 9.30am-7pm, Weekends 9.30am-6.30pm.
Weekends, school holidays and after 2pm term time Over 3s £4.95, Under 3s £3.95, Active babies £1.20, free for non-playing babies.
Term time up to 2pm Toddler activity mornings 10-11.30am £4.50, Play time 11.30am-2pm £3.50. 'Play and meal' deals are on offer and do make sense if you're planning on eating.
Unit 1a, Albany Trading Estate, Albany Road, Chorlton, Manchester M21 0AZ
Tel: 0161 881 4433 www.headoverheelsplay.co.uk

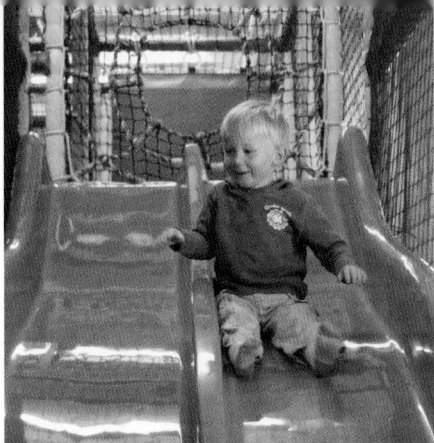

Run of the Mill is another favourite in the indoor play field.

The Jungle has got good equipment and is nice and clean. Highlights are probably the four-lane bumpy slide, which is long and fast, and the two enclosed trampolines. There are two small areas for under threes, a ball pit and an enclosed helter skelter slide. Sandwiches, toasties and soup are offered plus good coffee. Seating areas are on two levels. Friday from 4-6pm is Disco Night, where the lights are turned down and the music turned up. Free arts and crafts sessions are held twice a day on Tuesdays and Wednesdays for the under fives during term time.
Daily 10am-6pm.
Mon-Fri (term time) 10am-3.30pm £4 for the first child/£3 for additional children – includes a free tea or coffee plus juice. After school, weekends and school holidays £4.50 for all children. Under 1s free at all times.
12 Chetham Court, Calver Road, Winwick Quay, Warrington WA2 8RF
Tel: 01925 659995 www.thejungle.uk.net

PARENT AND BABY OR TODDLER GROUPS

Unfortunately the space allocated within this book is not sufficient to provide a review of the numerous and excellent Parent and Baby/Toddler Groups held all over Greater Manchester. In our opinion, they play a vital part in surviving the pre-school years and we would recommend seeking out one or more in your area. The best port of call for the most up to date information, is your health visitor or local NCT group (see page 85).

Initially arriving at a church hall (where many of these groups are held) to be greeted by a bunch of strangers who all appear to be in cliques, finding a few playmats on the floor and a selection of toys that you would not put out for your dog, never mind your new baby, can be intimidating and off-putting. But with a few deep breaths and a little patience you will mostly discover the groups are non-denominational, the toys are sterile in comparison to little Tarquin chewing the toilet brush at home, that your baby will adore the interaction with other babies and

before you know it, you will have your own little clique.

The cost of attendance is usually around £1 per visit. Most are run on a 'drop-in' basis but you may find there is a waiting list for some and a requirement to pay per term. For your pound, refreshments tend to be provided for toddlers and you'll get a cup of tea or coffee and one too many biscuits. Whilst the biscuits might not do much for your post-pregnancy figure, getting out of the house and meeting up with someone else who hasn't had more than three hours' sleep in the last six months and discovering their baby screams more than yours can do a great deal for your mental state.

The toddler groups offer more than a few playmats and rattles. A regular Tuesday session we attend includes age appropriate toys, an art area, a playdough table, indoor bikes and a slide, with a singing slot at the end. Hopefully lasting friendships for both yourself and your children can be made by attending a parent toddler group, as is the case with the mums behind this book.

Kiddie Chaos is set in a huge industrial unit with around 50 tables for parents. It does get busy at the weekends and when parties are on, but the size of the play area means there's room for everybody. There's a four-lane astro slide, enclosed football pitch, exercise balls, climbing rope, trampoline and excellent enclosed floor to ceiling slide. There is also a small area for babies by the under fives zone, which contains a two-lane slide.

Food includes fishfingers, chips, beans, sausages, pizzas for around £3.25.
Mon-Fri 9.30am-2pm Tot Time (during term time only) £2, 2-6pm £3.50, Under 1s 50p Weekends and School Holidays £3.95, Under 1s 50p
Mon-Sun 10am-6pm.
Unit 1, Gorton Crescent, Windmill Lane Industrial Estate, Denton M34 3RB
Tel: 0161 320 7774 www.kiddie-chaos.co.uk

Little Monsters Mayhem is a very well thought out centre. Its three areas contain a baby part with soft shapes, mirrors and wall activities; an under threes section with slide and ball pit and the main larger area for older children with a three-lane astro slide, zip wires, climbing walls and a perspex car you can pretend to drive. What does catch your eye is a mini-circuit with scooters that adjust to become ride-ons. There are comfy leather sofas and lots of tables and chairs. The café menu is simple but healthy with toasties, sandwiches and jackets. For £2.90 you can get a platter which includes a choice of sandwiches, fruit, crisps, yoghurt and drink.
Mon-Sat 9.30am-6pm, Sun 10am-6pm.
Child £3.75, Under 1s free.
Station Approach, 632 Liverpool Road, Irlam M44 5AD
Tel: 0161 775 5515 www.littlemonstersmayhem.co.uk

Mischief Makers is impressively clean with a small baby section; a toddler zone with a ball pit, giant wobbly skittles and a low slung circular swing; and an area for 5-11year olds which has a three-run astro slide, helter skelter and basketball court amongst other things, laid out over four levels. The menu's not as extensive as other places we visited but is adequate and low cost. Baby jars are available and cost 90p. Pizza and play sessions are run Mondays 4-6pm where you get playtime, pizza, juice and ice-cream included in the price of £5.75.
Daily term time 10am-4pm, holiday time 10am-6pm.
Over 2s £4.25, Under 2s £2.50, Under 1s free (if with paying child).
No 1 The Pavilions, Bridgefold Road, Rochdale OL11 5BX Tel: 01706 653 656 www.mischiefmakersltd.co.uk

Party and Play Funhouse is huge and being housed in a massive warehouse, allows the parents' seating area to be in the middle of all the equipment so you can pretty much see your child playing anywhere in the room. The giant doors of the building are actually fully retractable, so in good weather they're opened

POTTERY STUDIOS

Pottery Studios are a great place to visit. They're particularly good if you're stuck for present ideas for relatives or if perhaps the weather's off and you fancy letting your child's artistic temperament bloom. For the unitiated in the world of children's pottery painting, the studios are set up with a selection of white ware – from simple mugs and plates to piggy banks, letter racks and teapots. You purchase whatever you'd like, then you or your child paint it in the studio; you leave your artwork to be glazed and fired, then collect it in a few days. Prices vary to suit everyone's pocket; they usually range from around £5-£25. For a special memento, a lot of my friends had their baby's hand or footprint put onto a white tile or plate together with name and date – it's very effective. In the list below, you'll find most of the studios have refreshments on site and some are even linked with soft play areas.

The Art Café
Mon-Fri 10.30am-6pm, Sat 10.30am-6pm, Sun 11am-5pm.
2 Century House, Ashley Road, Hale, Cheshire WA15 9SF
Tel: 0161 929 6886

Brookside Pottery
Next to miniature railway – see page 25
Weekends 11am-4pm (sometimes Weds – please check)
Brookside Garden Centre, Macclesfield Road, Poynton
Cheshire SK12 1BY Tel: Liz 07946 637 499

The Ceramic Art Café at Tumble Jungle
Daily approx 11am-6pm (best to phone ahead).
Tumble Jungle (soft play centre), 168 Chorley New Road,
Horwich, Lancs BL6 5QW Tel: 01204 696158

Crackpots Ceramics Café (also has soft play area)
Mon-Fri 10am-5pm, Sat 10am-5.30pm, Sun 11am-4pm.
Unit 8, The Bridge Shopping Centre, Knutsford Road,
Latchford, Warrington WA4 1JR Tel: 01925 638 313
www.crackpotscafe.co.uk

Design a Pot Studios
Mon and Tues 2-6pm, Thurs 11am-7pm, Fri 11am-6pm,
Sat 10am-6pm, Sun 11am-5pm (during school holidays
studio open daily 10am-6pm).
16-18 Bank Street, Bolton BL1 1TS
Tel: 01204 365986 www.designapotstudios.co.uk

Funizuz Play Centre
Daily 10am-6pm (pottery shop within the soft play centre).
Brookfield Road Industrial Estate, Cheadle SK8 2PN
Tel: 0161 491 6611 www.funizuz.co.uk

Pottery Corner
Tues-Sat 10am-6pm and Sun 11am-5pm.
34 Beech Road, Chorlton, Manchester M21 9EL
Tel: 0161 882 0010 www.potterycorner.co.uk

Wild Orchid at The Studio, The Bluebell (within a florist).
Term time Mon 12-2.30pm, Thurs and weekends 11am-4pm.
Holidays open daily 11am-4pm (advisable to phone first).
The Bluebell, Stockport Road, Gee Cross, Hyde, Cheshire
SK14 5EZ Tel: 07968 102217 www.wild-orchids.org.uk

CLASSES AND ACTIVITIES

Activities

BABY LOVES DISCO

If you fancy dancing to some great club classics rather than the more traditional nursery rhymes, then this is the place for you. After a warm welcome from staff who'll safely store your pushchair, you head downstairs into Pure nightclub. It's like descending into a big children's party, except there's no birthday girl, the music isn't too loud – you can hear yourself speak – and the lights are not too dark to scare children. I was pleasantly surprised at the amount of dads there and though many had no doubt been coerced they looked like they were enjoying themselves. For the children, there were balloons, shakers, scarves, face painting and an unlimited supply of healthy party snacks. For the parents there was an adult only bar and a free massage for the more stressed out parents.

Upstairs, for babies and those not so keen on the music and lights, there is a chill-out room with comfy sofas, books, baby toys and mats.

The changing station is downstairs with free nappies and baby wipes. The nightclub apparently gets a triple clean before any babies come through the door. Although an expensive afternoon, it's great fun so why not take advantage of our offer on page 94 and strut your stuff.
Monthly Sunday afternoon 2-5pm. Admission: £8 per walking person, crawlers free. Age: 6 months to 7 years.
Pure, The Printworks, 27 Withy Grove, Manchester M4 2BS www.babylovesdisco.co.uk

CHILL FACTORE

If you're looking for something a little out of the ordinary, check out the Chill Factore. Real snow indoors all year round means a winter wonderland really is permanently on our doorstop here in Manchester.

Once inside you'll find all the trappings of an alpine village. Mums can get a fix of some delicious hot chocolate from the bars overlooking the piste, while the children will be looking wide-eyed at all that snow. Next to the main slope is the 'Snow Play Area', which is filled with mounds of real snow and pretend trees with a mini wooden chalet to play in. It's designed for 2-10 year olds and contains soft-play toys like polar bears and penguins.

This is great fun and entirely unique within the area, but the most obvious point to make is that it is of course extremely cold, so dress accordingly (gloves are essential). You can hire out suits and gloves at a cost of £3 if you pre-book or £5 on the day. Helmets, again compulsory, are supplied and are included in the entry fee.

Private ski-lessons are available for those aged three years and up – £35 for half an hour, with £7 for any extra friends you want to join the lesson. Saturday mornings also have group ski lessons – the Kindergarten Club is for those aged 4-6 years old. Tubing is available for children over four, and there's a luge for the over eights.
Snow Play is open Mon-Fri 10am-10pm and weekends 9am-10pm. Adults £1, Children £5 (parental supervision required at all times).
Chill Factore, Trafford Way, Trafford Quays Leisure Village, Manchester M41 7JA Tel: 0161 749 2222 www.chillfactore.com

up making this a great venue even on sunny days. All the usual climbing structures can be found here – a four-lane wavy slide, a curly tree slide and perspex tunnels to crawl through. There's a good toddler area for under fours which has the bonus of Little Tikes Cars. There are also two enclosed trampolines and a climbing wall. The café menu is quite large and includes a tasty sounding breakfast. Lunchtime adult food ranges from a Greek platter to cheesy nachos whilst the children's menu has such meals such as salmon fishcakes, sausage and chips and lunchboxes from £3.10.
Mon-Thurs 9.30am-7pm; Fri-Sun 9.30am-6pm.
Mon-Sun Over 1s £4.49, Under 1s 50p .
Weekends Over 1s £4.99, Under 1s £1 (free if with paying sibling).
South Westregen House, Off Great Bank Road, Wingates Industrial Park, Westhoughton, Bolton BL5 3XB Tel: 01942 818 195/ 01942 816 736
www.partyandplayfunhouse.co.uk

Planet Play When you walk in to Planet Play you are faced with a large three-level play frame with a tunnel slide into an incredibly deep ball pit. This area is aimed at older children and also includes air-powered ball-guns, a scary spook room and zip wires. There are two other sections: one for under sixes which includes a fast slide, ball pit and a big cooking pot style swing; and one for under threes, which although quite small does have a little house and small ball pit. There are also lots of ride-on vehicles. The café menu is very extensive.
Daily Mon-Sun 10am-6.30pm.
Over 18 months Mon-Fri before 2pm £3.50, after 2pm £3.75, weekends and holidays £4.25. 12-18 months Mon-Fri before 2pm £2, after 2pm £2.50, weekends and holidays £2.75. Under 12 months free.
2 Bradshaw Street, Heywood, OL10 1PN
Tel: 01706 627627 www.planetplay.net

Rumble in the Jungle is based in an old building with a car park at the back and does not feel as inviting as it might. You can leave your pushchair

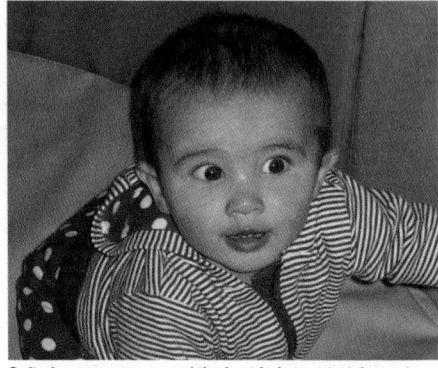
Soft play areas are one of the best indoor entertainment options for under fives.

CLASSES AND ACTIVITIES

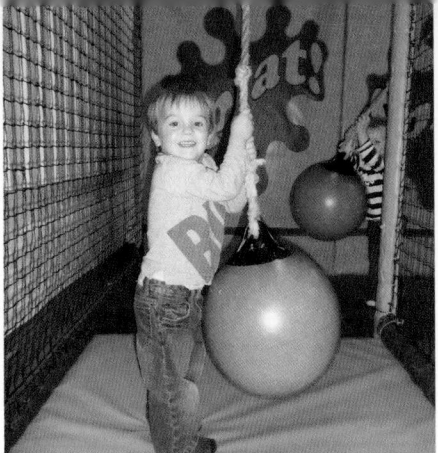

Run of the Mill is specifically geared towards the younger set.

Activities

Run of the Mill is really well thought out. We especially like this play centre because it seems particularly geared towards the younger set and isn't overwhelming like some of the others (despite the fact that it's big – over 10,000 square feet). There are up and over climbs, leapfrog trampettes, wavy slides, an enclosed sports pitch, sky gliders, a giant ball zone and a junior traverse wall amongst many other things! For toddlers, there is a sweet little vehicle area with various ride-ons as well as a specially designed playframe for under fours, which also includes a baby playpen).

Another outstanding feature is the menu – Mark's the chef and prides himself on delivering freshly prepared, home-cooked food of a very high standard. We enjoyed a Lebanese influenced mezze, panini and kid's sole goujons.
Daily 10am-6pm. Under 1s £1, Over 3s £4.25, Under 3s £3.50, Parent and Toddler sessions Mon-Fri 10am-2pm (term time) £3 including juice and a biscuit. Good after school meal deals (term time) on offer. Pear Mill, Stockport Road West, Bredbury, Stockport, Cheshire SK6 2BP Tel: 0161 494 7137 www.runofthemill.co.uk

downstairs as the play area is on the first floor. The whole facility is aimed at under fives. It has three small areas; a two-level climbing frame with tunnel slide and small ball pit; an under threes play pit with soft shapes and wall activities plus a ride-on car area. We really like the idea of an under fives only centre, but feel it could do with an overhaul as it's looking a bit tired. Children's meals include a lunchbox or chicken nuggets/hot dog and chips for £2.30.
Mon-Fri 9.30am-5.30pm, Weekends 10am-5.30pm. Over 1s £3.20, Under 1s £1.20. Hallam Mill, Hallam St, Stockport, Cheshire SK2 6PT Tel: 0161 477 8438 www.rumbleinthejungle.co.uk

Slide and Seek is set in a huge warehouse with a vast café area. The junior section is four levels high with a four-lane astro slide and also contains a basketball area with nets. Toddlers have their own two-lane slide and a ball pit; there are also Little Tike cars in a circuit and a kitchen area. There is a

CLASSES AND ACTIVITIES

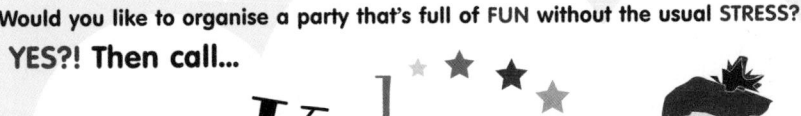
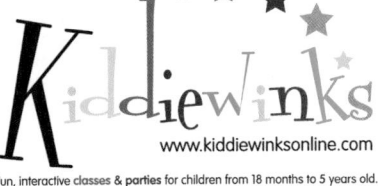
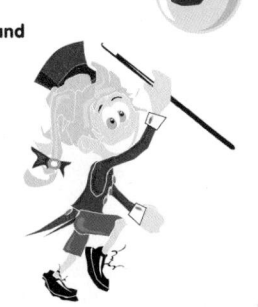

Activities

baby zone with soft shapes and panel games. Children's meals start at £1.50 for pasta. There is also a pick and mix selection of chicken nuggets, fishfingers, chips, carrot sticks, beans and juice for £3.50 or lunchboxes for the same price.
Mon-Fri 9.30am-6pm, Weekends 10am-6pm. Toddler activity mornings during term time Mon-Fri 9.30am-2pm £3.50, including a free drink and snack, Under 1s free. After 2pm, school holidays and weekends, Over 3s £4.50, Under 3s £3.50, Under 12 months free.
Unit A, SK14 Industrial Park, Broadway, Hyde SK14 4QF
Tel: 0161 366 8080 www.slideandseek.co.uk

Snakes and Slides is a large soft play centre with a baby and toddler area. There is a wide variety of play equipment for older toddlers and children including a traverse wall, a football zone and four-lane astro slide. The café seating area is directly between the play equipment and the entrance. A good selection of food is available.
Mon-Sat 9.30am-6pm, Sun 10am-5pm. Mon-Fri term time, parent and toddler sessions £3.50 before 2pm; after 2pm Mon-Fri, weekend and school holidays £4.50 for the first child, £4 for any other child after, under six months free.
Unit 3, Rule Business Park, Grimshaw Lane, Middleton M24 2AE Tel: 0161 653 1221
www.snakesandslides.co.uk

CINEMAS

Parent Baby Screenings

We've found two cinemas that offer special parent and baby screenings, Nappy Mondays at the Apollo in Altrincham and Newbies at the Odeon in both the Trafford Centre and Rochdale. This is great as it takes away all the embarrassment of watching a film with a screaming baby in tow, but still probably not the time to practice controlled crying! Currently running once a week, there is no choice of film, but it is usually one of the most recent releases. Legally it has to be a 12A rating or below, as children are in the audience. You pay only for the adult, at normal cinema entrance price.

Altrincham Apollo is a fairly small cinema and was very quiet for our visit – there were only about 15-20 mums with offspring. Mostly they were babies on laps, but there were some toddlers. There is no official upper age limit for children, but older ones tend to get bored by the end. The volume is a bit lower and lighting is kept slightly up throughout the film which allows for feeding etc. Bottle and baby food heating duty was taken on by the popcorn counter staff. Pushchairs are allowed right in to the cinema which makes life a lot easier. During showings at the Trafford Centre Cinema, pushchairs need to be left outside in the office and collected after the film, which can be awkward if you have a sleeping baby.

Overall there is a very relaxed atmosphere, which enables everyone to enjoy the chance to get out and watch a film. Whenever I have been, the babies present have all been remarkably well behaved, in fact I am always surprised at how little noise they make, and how little they disrupt the viewing. Baby changing facilities are available.
Nappy Monday Mon 12noon Adult £5.80, Babies free.
Apollo Altrincham, Denmark St, Altrincham WA14 2WG
Tel: 0871 220 6000 www.apollocinemas.co.uk
Newbies Tues 11.30am Adult £5.10, Toddlers up to four free.
Odeon Trafford Centre, 201 The Dome, The Trafford Centre, Manchester M17 8DF
Newbies Wed 11.20am Adult £5.65, Toddlers up to four free.
Odeon Rochdale, Sandbrook Park, Sandbrook Way, Lancs OL11 1RY
Tel: 0871 22 44 007 www.odeon.co.uk/fanatic/newbies/

Kids Cinema

Every weekend most cinemas host screenings for children – ideal if you haven't been to the cinema with them before and aren't sure if they're going to like it. In most cases one adult is free per child or there is a nominal charge. They are not always the latest releases, but the majority of under fives don't seem to care what they're watching. This is a great rainy day activity and if you don't get too caught up buying popcorn and drinks, it doesn't cost the earth.
Apollo Altrincham
Apollo Kids Club Sat 10.30am Adult and Child £1.50
Denmark St, Altrincham WA14 2WG
Tel: 0871 220 6000 www.apollocinemas.co.uk
Cineworld
Movies for Juniors Sat 10am Adult and Child £1 each.
Ashton Leisure Park, Fold Way, Off Lord Sheldon Way, Ashton-under-Lyne OL7 0PG
The Valley, 15 Eagley Brook Way, Bolton BL1 8TS
4 Grand Central Square, Wellington Road South, Stockport SK1 3TA
Movies for Juniors Sat 10.20am, 10.30am and 10.40am Adult and Child £1 each.
Parrs Wood Entertainment Centre, Wilmslow Road, Didsbury M20 5PG
Tel: 0871 200 2000 www.cineworld.co.uk
Odeon
Kids Club Weekends 11am Child £2.45, Adults free.
The Printworks, 27 Withy Grove, Manchester M4 2BS
The Trafford Centre, Manchester M17 8DF
Kids Club Weekends 11am Child £2.50, Adults free.
Sandbrook Park, Sandbrook Way, Lancs OL11 1RY
Tel: 0871 22 44 007 www.odeon.co.uk/fanatic/kids
Vue
Kids AM Weekends 10.30am Child £1.70, Adults free.
Lowry Outlet Mall, The Quays, Salford Quays, Salford M50 3AH
Middlebrook Leisure Park, The Link Way (Off Mansel Way), Horwich, Bolton BL6 6JA
Park 66, Pilsworth Road, Bury BL9 8RS
Tel: 08712 240 240 www.myvue.com

Most children love swimming and the earlier they start, the better, plus it's great exercise for you too. Below is a list of toddler times and swimming lessons available in the Greater Manchester area.

Swimming Pools

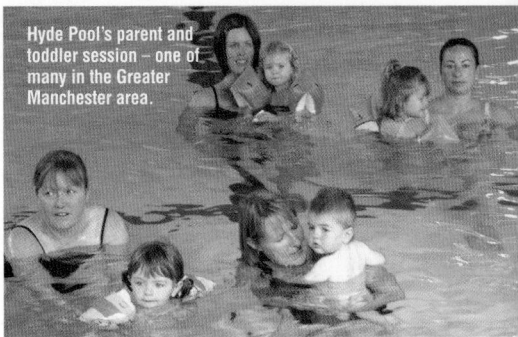

Hyde Pool's parent and toddler session – one of many in the Greater Manchester area.

BOLTON

Farnworth Leisure Centre Six-lane main pool and a teaching pool. Parent and Tots Sessions from 6 months to 5 years held Mon, Wed & Fri 12-1.00pm and cost £2.95 per session. There's no need to book; floats and toys are available. It's life-guarded session, no instructor.
Swim Life swimming lessons available from 3 years. A 10-week course costs £42.50, classes available Mon-Fri and Sat mornings.
Family swim main pool: Sat 9am-2pm, Sun 9am-4pm.
Family swim small pool: Sat 1-3.30pm, Sun 9am-3.30pm.
Adult £2.95, Under 16s £1.60, Under 3s free.
Brackley Street, Farnworth, Bolton BL4 9DZ
Tel: 01204 334477 www.boltonleisure.com

Horwich Leisure Centre Main pool, teaching pool and crèche. Parent and Tots sessions Tues-Thurs 12-12.30pm or 12.30-1pm for children aged 6 months to 5 years. It's instructor led with floats and toys and costs £2.95.
Swim Life swimming lessons available from 3 years. A 10-week course costs £42.50, classes available Mon-Fri and Sat mornings.
Family swim main pool: Mon 3-6.30pm, Tues-Fri 3-7pm, Sat 9am-2pm and Sun 9am-4pm.
Family swim small pool: Mon-Fri 3-4pm, Mon Weds and Fri 6-7.30pm, Sat 12.30-3.30pm, Sun 9am-4pm.
Adult £2.95, Under 16s £1.60, Under 4s free. Café.
Victoria Road, Horwich, Bolton BL6 5PY
Tel: 01204 334426 www.boltonleisure.com

LadyBridge Leisure Centre One main pool with family swim Sat 1-2pm and Sun 9.30am-1pm. Swim Life swimming lessons available from 3 years. A 10-week course costs £42.50, classes available Mon-Fri and Sat mornings.
Adult £2.95, Under 16s £1.60, Under 3s free.
New York Road, Deane, Bolton BL3 4NG
Tel: 01204 334432 www.boltonleisure.com

Westhoughton Leisure Centre Two pools with Parent and Tots Swim lessons on Thurs 1-2pm suitable for children aged 6 months to 5 years. Floats and toys available and it costs £2.95 per session.
Swim Life swimming lessons available from 3 years. A 10-week course costs £42.50, classes available Mon-Fri and Sat mornings.
Family swim in small pool: Sat 1.30-4pm, Sun 9am-4pm.
Adult £2.95, Under 16s £1.60, Under 3s free.
Bolton Road, Westhoughton, Bolton BL5 3BZ
Tel: 01942 634810 www.boltonleisure.com

Sharples Leisure Centre One main pool. Swim Life swimming lessons available from 3 years. A 10-week course costs £42.50, classes available Mon-Fri and Sat mornings.
Aqua Natal Classes Thurs 6.30-7.30pm £3.60 per session.
Family swim Mon-Wed 5.30-7.30pm, Thurs 5.30-6.30pm, Fri 6-8pm, Sat 1-2pm, Sun 9.30am-3pm.
Adult £2.95, Under 16s £1.60, Under 3s free.
Hill Cot Road, Sharples, Bolton BL1 8SN
Tel: 01204 334224 www.boltonleisure.serco.com

Turton Leisure Centre One main pool. Swim Life swimming lessons available from 3 years. A 10-week course costs £42.50, classes available Mon-Fri and Sat mornings.
Family swim Mon 6.30-8.30pm, Thurs 5-7pm, Fri 5.30-7pm, Sun 9.30-11.45am.
Adult £2.95, Under 16s £1.60, Under 3s free.
Chapeltown Road, Bromley Cross, Bolton BL7 9LT
Tel: 01204 334440 www.boltonleisure.serco.com

BURY

Castle Leisure Centre Three pools and Parent and Toddler drop-in sessions with toys Mon & Weds 1-2pm, Sat 11.30am-12.30pm. Mother and Toddler drop-in sessions with toys are Weds 12-1pm. All cost £3.00 for parent/mother and toddler.
Swimming lessons available for 3-5 year olds, a 10-week course costs £42 (parents not in water).
The Baby Pool is open daily but times vary. Café.
Bolton Street, Bury BL9 0EZ
Tel: 0161 253 6513 www.bury.gov.uk

Radcliffe Pool & Fitness Centre No family swim, but advised to come with under fives in term-time when it's quieter and you can usually use the baby pool, which has floats and a small slide: Mon, Tues, Fri 10.30am-4pm; Weds 9am-1.30pm; Thurs 11.30am-1.30pm; Sat 11am-3.30pm and Sun 8am-1.30pm.
Adults £2.80, Under 16s £1.40, Under 5s 60p.
Swimming lessons available from 3yrs (phone for details). Family changing room currently being built. Creche on site Mon-Fri 10am-3pm.
Green Street, Radcliffe M26 3ED
Tel: 0161 253 7814 www.bury.gov.uk

Ramsbottom Pool and Fitness Centre One pool. Mother and Baby sessions held Weds 9.30-10.30am. It's run with a teacher on a drop-in basis and costs £2.90.
Swimming lessons for under 5s (a 10-week course costs £42) available Mon and Weds afternoon, Tues and Fri mornings, weekdays after school, Sat mornings and Sun afternoons.
Adults £2.80, Under 16s £1.40, Under 5s 60p.
Porritt Way, Ramsbottom, Bury BL0 0PT
Tel: 0161 253 7292 www.bury.gov.uk

CLASSES AND ACTIVITIES

Swimming pools

Manchester Aquatics Centre Manchester Aquatics has excellent pools! The large baby pool (complete with jacuzzi and elephant slides) is open Mon and Weds 9am-5.30pm; Tues, Thurs-Sun 9am-8pm. There are specific Family Sessions held in the baby pool at weekends 9am-1pm and this is for under eights only. The other thing to bear in mind is that generally speaking the baby pool (which is open to all visitors, not just little ones) is quieter during school times. The next pool is the 23m, which is quite a shallow pool allocated for 'social swimming' so children are happily allowed in this Mon and Weds 9am-5.30pm; Tues, Thurs and Fri 9am-8pm and weekends 9am-6pm.
Adult £3.10, Under 16s £1.90, Under 5s free.
Swimming lessons available from 6 months. A 10-week course costs £33, classes available weekend mornings. Up to the age of 3 adults must be in the water too.
There are four family changing rooms and you can lock your pram away at reception when you arrive. Café.
2 Booth Street East, Ardwick, Manchester M13 9SS
Tel: 0161 275 9450 www.manchestersportandleisure.org

Abraham Moss Leisure Centre Baby Pool open 10-11am on Saturday (£2.40 for parents, free for babies but no toys). General swimming with children in the main pool is all the time except first thing in the mornings and 12-1pm when it's adults only. You can buy a family ticket for £6.
Swimming lessons available from 4 years. A 10-week course costs £35, classes available Mon and Weds eve.
Crescent Road, Crumpsall, Manchester M8 5UF
Tel: 0161 720 7622 www.manchester.gov.uk

Broadway Leisure Centre One main pool. Parent and baby sessions Fri 1pm, 1.30pm and 2pm (10-week course costs £35). Family swim for under fives weekends 12-1pm (no toys). Children are allowed in the pool at all times except adult only sessions Mon-Thurs 9-10pm and Weds 7-8pm.
Adults £2.40, Under 16s £1.50, Under 5s free.
New Moston, Manchester M40 0LN
Tel: 0161 681 1060 www.manchester.gov.uk

Chorlton Leisure Centre Family swim (with toys) are every Sun 10-11am and 12-1pm (allowed two under fours with one adult).
Swimming lessons available from 6 months to three and a half years old. Classes Sat mand weekday mornings. Parents must be in the pool too. Swimming lessons also available from four and a half years old on Mon, Weds, Thurs after school and Sat mornings (10-week courses for both cost £35).
Aqua Natal is a drop-in on Tuesday 12-1pm, new mums can pop along and leave their babies poolside whilst they swim. Midwives from St Marys Hospital are around as well. Changing cabins are poolside so baby changing limited to changing mats.
Adults £2.40, Under 16s £1.50, Under 5s free.
Manchester Road, Chorlton, Manchester M21 9PQ
Tel: 0161 861 0790 www.manchester.gov.uk

Forum Leisure Two pools. Parent and Toddler session for under 5s (no toys) in the small pool Mon-Fri 12-1pm (£2.30).
Swimming lessons available for over 4s. A 10-week course costs £35.
Family swims Tues 6-7.15pm, Thurs-Fri 6-7pm, weekends

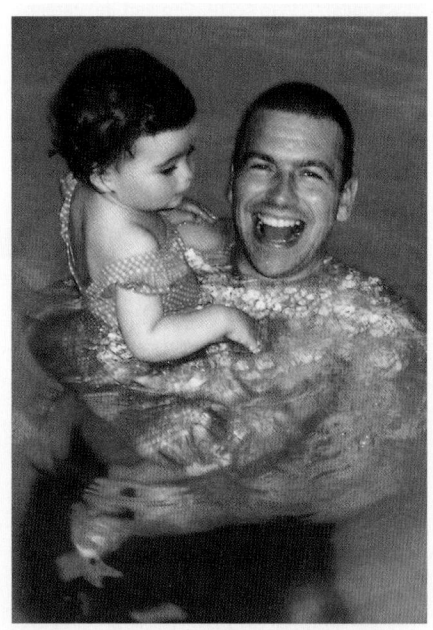

3-4pm. Small pool open at weekends, phone for times.
Adults £2.40, Under 16s £1.50, Under 5s free. Café.
Forum Centre, Forum Square, Wythenshawe, Manchester M22 5RX Tel: 0161 935 4020 www.manchester.gov.uk

Levenshulme Swimming Pools Parent and toddler drop-in sessions with toys are Weds 12-1pm and Sat 1-2pm. Costs £2.40 (£1.90 with Manchester Leisure pass). Children are welcome in the pools at all other times except adult only sessions which are Mon-Fri 12-1pm and 8-9.45pm.
Adults £2.40 (£1.90 with Manchester Leisure pass), Under 16s £1.50, Under 5s free, Family Swim £6.
Changing cubicles and changing table are poolside.
Barlow Road, Levenshulme, Manchester M19 3HE
Tel: 0161 224 4370 www.manchester.gov.uk

Miles Platting Swimming Pool Swimming lessons available from 6 months. A 10-week course costs £33.
Family swim every Saturday 10.30am-12pm.
£2.40 for adults and under 5s go free. You can also use the family pool Thurs 4.30-7pm, Fri 3.30-6pm (no toys).
Varley Street, Miles Platting, Manchester M40 8EE
Tel: 0161 205 8939
www.info.milesplattingpool@leisure.serco.com

Moss Side Leisure Centre Parent and toddler sessions for under 5s in the heated baby pool, Mon 12-1pm, 3.30-7pm; Tues 5.30-6.30pm; Weds 12-1pm, 3.30-4pm; Fri 12-1pm, 4-7pm; Sat 12-2pm; Sun 10-2pm. Costs £2.40.
Adult £2.40, Under 16s £1.50, Under 5s free.
Swimming lessons available up to 3 years. A 10-week course costs £35, classes available Tues and Thurs 12-12.30pm. Parents must be in the pool too.
Moss Lane East, Moss Side, Manchester M15 5NN
Tel: 0161 226 5015 www.manchester.gov.uk

Ivy Bank Swimming School, Prestwich

A real hidden gem… Privately owned and managed, and looking from the outside like a bungalow with a conservatory attached, Ivy Bank is a small pool (7m by 3.5m) that can be hired out for parties or simply by a group of parents who want a pool to themselves. There is also a comprehensive schedule of swimming lessons from three years old that cost £42 for seven lessons (run daily after school and at weekends 9.30am-12 noon). Also Aquanauts runs kiddie classes from birth upwards at Ivy Bank two days a week (www.aquanauts.uk.com).

If you would like to hire out the pool privately it costs around £6 for two adults and one child. For two adults and two children it's £7.50 – there is no lifeguard.

If you want to hire the pool for a party it's around £40 for one hour with a lifeguard and inflatables. There are two changing cubicles by the side of the pool (no baby changing so bring your own mats) with a toilet in each.

The diary for bookings is kept just one week in advance so plenty of scope to get a slot! Parents who've been really rave about it saying it's perfect for toddlers.

A great place to book all year round but a real treat in the summer months! Vending machine available.
31 Grosvenor Street, Prestwich, Manchester M25 1ES
Tel: 0161 773 2629

North City Family and Fitness Centre

Parent, Babies and Toddlers up to six years with toys Tues 1-2pm. Cost £2.30. Public swim is generally every day 3.30pm onwards. Family swim weekends 9-11am.
Adults £2.40, Under 16s £1.50, Under 6s free.
Upper Conran Street, Harpurhey, Manchester M9 4DA
Tel: 0161 277 1900 www.manchester.gov.uk

Withington Swimming Pool and Fitness Centre

Family swim Sunday 10-11.30am (no toys provided).
Adults £2.40, Under 16s £1.50, Under 5s free.
Changing cabins are poolside with family changing area.
30 Burton Road, Withington M20 3EB
Tel: 0161 445 1973 www.leisurebookings.net

OLDHAM

Crompton Pool

Parent and baby sessions (with instructor and sing-song) Weds 9.30-11.30am £3.80 and Thurs (no instructor or singing) 9.30-11.30am £3.20. For under fives.
Farrow Street, Shaw OL2 8NW
Tel: 0161 621 3260 www.ocll.co.uk

Failsworth Sport Centre

Parent and baby drop-in sessions on Tues 11.30am-12.30pm. Costs £3.80 and is for under 5s.
Brierley Avenue, Failsworth, Manchester M35 9HA
Tel: 0161 621 3240 www.ocll.co.uk

Glodwick Pool

Parent and baby drop-in sessions on Weds 10-11.30am with toys and music (actual class starts at 10.30am). Costs £3.80 and is for under 4s.
Nugget Street, Glodwick OL4 1BN
Tel: 0161 621 3280 www.ocll.co.uk

Oldham Sports Centre

Parent and baby sessions with toys (drop-in for up to two and a half years) on Weds 10.30-11.30am

and Fri 11.30-12.30am. £3.80 in the small pool.
Aqua Tots swimming lessons available from two and a half years. A 10-week course costs £46, classes available Mon-Thurs after school, Fri 5.30-7.30pm and Sat 9am-1pm.
Adults £3.80, Under 18s £1.60, Under fours free. Family ticket £7.20. Pram-locks. Café.
Lord Street, Oldham, Manchester OL1 3HA
Tel: 0161 621 3220 www.ocll.co.uk

Royton Sports Centre

Parent and baby drop-in sessions on Thurs and Sat 12-12.45pm. Costs £3.80.
There is a crèche facility Tues, Weds and Thurs mornings.
Park Street, Royton OL2 6QW
Tel: 0161 621 3250 www.ocll.co.uk

Saddleworth Pool

Parent and baby drop-in sessions on Tues 12-1pm with toys. Costs £3.20 and is for under fours.
Station Road, Uppermill OL3 6HQ
Tel: 0161 621 3270 www.ocll.co.uk

ROCHDALE

Central Leisure Centre

Parent and baby drop-in sessions up to five years, with toys on Weds 12.30-1.30pm £3.30.
Adults £2.80, Under 16s £1.35, Under 5s 50p.
Entwisle Road, Rochdale OL16 2HZ
Tel: 01706 924213 www.link4life.org

Middleton Arena Leisure Centre

Parent and baby drop-in sessions with toys up to five years on Tues and Thurs 12-1.15pm, Sat 10.30am-1.30pm and 3-4pm (without instructor) £3.30.
Adults £2.80, Under 16s £1.35, Under 5s 50p.
Suffield Street, Middleton M24 1HB
Tel: 0161 662 4000 www.link4life.org

Heywood Sports Complex

Parent and baby drop-in sessions with toys up to five years on Mon and Tues 12.15-1.15pm (£3.30).
Adults £2.80, Under 16s £1.35, Under 5s 50p.
West Starkey Street, Heywood OL10 4TW
Tel: 01706 367212 www.link4life.org

SALFORD

Fit City Broughton Pool

Parent and toddler drop-in sessions in the baby pool Mon-Fri 12-1pm with toys and floats. Costs £3. Swimming lessons start from age four after school and on Saturday (there is a waiting list). Family swim Fri 5-6pm. Children are welcome at other times apart from Mon-Fri in the main pool 12-1pm when it's adult swim time.
Adults £3, Under 16s £1.60, Under 5s free.
Great Cheetham Street West, Salford M7 2DN
Tel: 0161 792 2847 www.leisureinsalford.info

Fit City Clarendon

Parent and baby free drop-in Weds 12-1pm. Fit City run their own parent and baby drop-ins (with toys) on Thurs 12-1pm, cost £3.
Swim City Kids Swimming lessons available for 3-5 year olds. A 10-week course costs £35, classes available Tues, Wed and Fri evenings and Sat mornings.
Adults £3, Under 16s £1.60, Under 5s free.
Liverpool Street, Salford M5 4LY
Tel: 0161 736 1494 www.salford.gov.uk

Fit City Eccles

Children welcome at all times except for adult only swims. Swimming courses available for three months to five years. Contact Fit City for details.

Swimming pools

Adults £3, Under 16s £1.60, Under 5s free.
Barton Lane, Eccles, Salford M30 0DD
Tel: 0161-787 7107 www.leisureinsalford.info

Fit City Irlam Pool Children welcome at all times when there aren't adult only swims.Swimming lessons available for 1-3 year olds on Mon and Weds.
Adults £3, Over 5s £1.60, Under 5s free.
Liverpool Road, Irlam M44 6BR
Tel: 0161 775 4134 www.salford.gov.uk/fitcity-ir.htm

Fit City Pendlebury Children welcome at all times when there aren't adult only swims.Swimming lessons available for three months to five years.
Adults £3, Under 16s £1.60, Under 5s free.
Cromwell Road, Swinton, Salford M27 2SZ
Tel: 0161 793 1750 www.leisureinsalford.info

Fit City Worsley Three pools and family swims on Fri 6.30-9.30pm and Sun 8.30am-12.30pm. The small pool is available Mon-Fri 12-1pm and 3-4pm (you can ask for floats) and Sun 12.30-4pm. Swimming lessons are available from three years.
Adults £3, Under 16s £1.60, Under 5s free, Family ticket £7.
Bridgewater Road, Walkden, Salford M28 3AB
Tel: 0161 790 2084 www.lesiureinsalford.info

STOCKPORT

Avondale Leisure and Target Fitness Centre Swim play drop-in session for parents and toddlers with toys and singing. Run by an instructor. Tues 11.05-11.40am and Sat 10.45am-11.15am (£2.95).
Family swim (with toys) Sun 10am-12pm.
Swimming lessons available from four years.
Adults £2.55, Under 16s £1.45, Under 3s free. Café.
Heathbank Road, Stockport SK3 0UP
Tel: 0161 477 4242 www.sportinstockport.com

Grand Central Pools
Mon-Fri 6.30am-10pm, Sat 7am-4.30pm, Sun 7am-10pm.
12 Grand Central Square, Wellington Road South,
Stockport SK1 3TA
Tel: 0161 474 7766 www.stockport.gov.uk

Hazel Grove Pools and Target Fitness Centre Swim play drop-in session for parents and toddlers with toys and singing. Run by a teacher it's not structured apart from a short singalong at the end. Mon 1.15-1.45pm; Thurs 10-10.30am, 10.30-11.30am, 1.15-1.45pm; Fri 1-1.30pm. Cost £2.95. After attending swim play the under fives progress to swim start and then swim link. These six-week courses cost £4.10 per lesson. Classes available Mon and Thurs. Family fun sessions in the small pool with toys are Sun 1.30-3.30pm.
Adults £2.55, Under 16s £1.45, Under 3s free.
The centre sells swim nappies at reception.
Jackson Lane, Hazel Grove SK7 5JW
Tel: 0161 439 5221 www.sportinstockport.com

Marple Swimming Pool Swim play drop-in session for parents and toddlers with toys and singing. Run by a teacher it's not structured apart from a short singalong at the end. Mon 1.15-1.45pm and Tues 2-2.30pm. Cost £2.50. After attending swim play the under fives progress to swim start and then swim link. These six-week courses cost £4.10 per lesson. Classes available Mon and Tues.
Public swimming weekends 7.30-11am.

Adults £2.55, Under 16s £1.45, Under 3s 75p.
Stockport Road, Marple, Stockport SK6 6AA
Tel: 0161 427 7070 www.sportinstockport.com

Target Fitness Cheadle Swim play drop-in session for parents and toddlers with toys and singing. Run by a teacher it's not structured apart from a short singalong at the end. Mon 9.15-9.45am, Tues and Thurs 12-12.30pm, Weds 10.15-11.15am and Sun 4-4.30pm. Cost £2.95. After attending swim play the under fives progress to swim start and then swim link. Cost £4.10 per lesson payable per term. Fun sessions (with inflatables and floats) in main and small pool on Sat 1.30-2.45pm.
Adults £2.55, Under 16s £1.45, Under threes free. Café area.
Soft play area in reception (£2 per child).
Shiers Drive, Cheadle, Stockport SK8 1JR
Tel: 0161 428 3216 www.sportinstockport.com

Target Fitness Romiley Two pools. Swim play drop-in session for parents and toddlers with toys and singing. Run by a teacher it costs £2.95. Mon 10.50-11.20am; Tues 9.45-10.15am, 10.15-10.45am, 10.45-11.15am; Thurs 11.30am-12pm; and Sat 12.45-1.15pm.
After attending swim play the under fives progress to swim start and then swim link. Payable per term it costs £4.10 per lesson. Classes available Tues and Sat mornings.
Adults £2.55, Under 16s £1.45, Under threes free.
Hole House Fold, Romiley, Stockport SK6 4BD
Tel: 0161 430 3437 www.sportinstockport.com

TRAFFORD

Altrincham Leisure Centre Parent and toddler drop-in session with toys in the small pool. Mon 12-1.30pm, Tues 12.30-1.15pm and Thurs 11.15am-12.15pm. Costs £3.30. Water confidence swimming lessons available for 0-3 year olds. A 10-week course costs £99, classes available Mon-Fri. Can be booked by calling 0161 657 0456 or www.enjoyswimming.org.
Swim well swimming lessons available for 3-4 half year olds. A 12-week course costs £49.75, classes available Mon and Thurs. Parents are also in the pool.
Small pool open Weds 2.30-7.45pm; Sat 2-5pm and Sun 9am-12.30pm and 2-5pm. Children are welcome in the main pool at other times apart from adult only swim times.
Adults £2.90, Under 16s £1.50, Under 5s 50p.
Oakfield Road, Altrincham, Cheshire WA15 8EW
Tel: 0161 926 3255 www.traffordleisure.co.uk

Partington Sports Village One main pool. Parent and toddler drop-in sessions on Mon 9.30-10.30am for up to five year olds, with a swimming teacher. Cost £2.90.
Dinkys class swimming lessons available from two and a half to three and a half years old. A 13-week course costs £49.75, classes available Fridays 3.30pm. Parents must be in the pool too.
Swim well swimming lessons available for three to four and a half year olds. A 13-week course costs £49.75.
Family fun sessions weekends 2-3pm.
Adults £2.90, Under 16s £1.50, Under 5s 50p.
Chapel Lane, Partington, Manchester M31 4ES
Tel: 0161 777 4222 www.traffordleisure.co.uk

Sale Leisure Centre Swimming lessons available from two and a half years old, with parents in the pool. Ducklings swimming lessons available from three and a half. A

Swimming pools

13-week course costs £49.75, classes Tues, Weds and Fri. Adults £2.90, Under 16s £1.50, Under 5s 50p. Café.
Broad Road, Sale, Manchester M33 2AL
Tel: 0161 905 5588 www.traffordleisure.co.uk

Stretford Leisure Centre Parent and toddler drop-in sessions, Tues and Weds 2-3.30pm, Thurs 10-11.30am term time only (£3.30). Also have drop-in dry play sessions called Tiny Ted upstairs Tues, Thurs and Fri 10-11.30am. These sessions cost £2.10 and include access to the soft play area there (open same times) and are held all year round (except the two-week Christmas period).
Swim well swimming lessons available from four years old. A 13-week course costs £49.75.
Adults £2.90, Under 16s £1.50, Under 5s 50p. Café.
Greatstone Road, Stretford, Manchester M32 0ZS
Tel: 0161 875 1414 www.traffordleisure.co.uk

Urmston Leisure Centre Parent and toddler drop-in sessions for under fives. Mon 2-3.45pm, Fri 10.30am-12.30pm, cost £3.30. Swimming lessons start from five years old.
Family fun swim Sat 2-3pm and Sun 9-12pm.
Adults £2.90, Under 16s £1.50, Under 5s 50p.
Bowfell Road, Urmston, Manchester M41 5RR
Tel: 0161 749 2570 www.traffordleisure.co.uk

Ashton Pools Two pools. Parent and child 'Ducklings' sessions held Mon, Weds and Fri 12-1.30pm. Designed to help introduce pre-school children to the water during semi-formal sessions with play, music and rhymes. Children achieve badges to mark their progress. Swimming lessons start from age five.
Adults £3.60, Under 16s £1.80, Under 5s 90p, Family ticket (two adults and three children) £7.50.
Water Street, Ashton-under-Lyne OL6 7AN
Tel: 0161 330 1179 www.tamesidesportstrust.com

The Copley Centre Two pools on site. Parent and child 'Ducklings' sessions Tues and Thurs 12.15-1.15pm and Sat 1-2pm. Duckling sessions help introduce pre-school children to the water during semi-formal sessions with play, music and rhymes. Children achieve badges to mark progress.
Adults £3.60, Under 16s £1.80, Under 5s 90p.
Family ticket (two adults and three children) £7.50.
Huddersfield Road, Stalybridge SK15 3ET
Tel: 0161 303 8118 www.tamesidesportstrust.com

Denton Pools Two pools. Parent and child (pre-schoolers) 'Two in a Tub' sessions Thurs 12-1pm and Tues (during term time) from 11.15am-12pm. Saturday 12.15pm-1.15pm family fun sessions with inflatables, floats and other equipment. Swimming lessons start from age five.
Adults £3.60, Under 16s £1.80, Under 5s 90p.
Family ticket (two adults and three children) £7.50.
Victoria Street, Denton M34 9GU
Tel: 0161 336 1900 www.tamesidesportstrust.com

Medlock Leisure Centre One main new pool. Parent and tot drop-in sessions with toys for under fives Fri 11.15am-12pm (term time) and Sun 12-1pm (£3.60 for adults and 90p for tots). 'Bubbles and Rhymes' sessions with books and bubbles are held monthly (£3.60 for adults and 90p for tots). Swimming lessons start from age five. Aquanatal sessions Tues 10-11am (term time) where a midwife is on hand.
Adults £3.60, Under 16s £1.80, Under 5s 90p.

Family ticket (two adults and three children) £7.50.
Garden Fold Way, Droylsden, Tameside M43 7XU
Tel: 0161 370 3070 www.tamesidesportstrust.com

Hyde Leisure Pool Currently closed for six months, expected to be open April/May 2009. Waves, bubbles, geysers, flume, lazy river plus more. Hyde is a free form pool where you can walk into the water from a gentle sloping beach-like approach, which is fantastic for toddlers. The centre is home to Wally Walrus. Wally sessions are exclusively for those with pre-school children under five. The emphasis is on basic water skills whilst playing games and having a singalong. Sessions take place every Tues 1-2.30pm term time and 9-10am during school holidays, on Fri 10-11.15am term time and 9-10am during school holidays and Wally's Saturday Club is 9.15-10.45am. Cost £4 (one adult and one child), under fives £1.10.
Adults £5, Under 16s £2.70, Under 5s £1.10.
Family ticket (two adults and three children) £12.90.
Walker Lane, Hyde, Tameside SK14 5PL
Tel: 0161 368 4057 www.tamesidesportstrust.com

Ashton Leisure Centre Parent and toddler sessions Tues 12-1pm and Fri 3.10-4pm (cost £3.70). A drop-in session for three to four year olds with an instructor is available on Thurs 12-1pm and costs £3.70. Swim well lessons available from age five. A 10-week course costs £37.
Adults £2.95, Under 16s free (if you purchase a lifestyle membership card for £1.50), Under 5s free.
Old Road, Ashton-in-Makerfield, Wigan WN4 9TP
Tel: 01942 720826 www.wlct.org

Hindley Pool Surestart runs drop-in parent and toddler sessions Mon-Weds at 1.10pm (you need to register). Swimming lessons available from age four. A 10-week course costs £37.
Adults £2.95, Under 16s free (if you purchase a lifestyle membership card for £1.50), Under 5s free.
Borsdane Road, Hindley WN2 3QN
Tel: 01942 255401 www.wlct.org

Howe Bridge Sports centre Two pools. Parent and toddler session on Thurs 9am-12pm and Fri 1.15-3.15pm. Costs £3.70. Swimming lessons available from age four. A 10-week course costs £37.
Adults £2.95, Under 16s free (if you purchase a lifestyle membership card for £1.50), Under 5s free.
Eckersley Fold Lane, Atherton, Manchester M46 0PJ
Tel: 01942 870403 www.wlct.org

Leigh Indoor Sports Centre One main pool. Parent and toddler sessions Tues and Thurs 1.30-2.30pm. Swimming lessons available from age five (10-week course £37).
Adults £2.95, Under 16s free (if you purchase a lifestyle membership card for £1.50), Under 5s free.
Sale Way, Leigh Sports Village, Leigh, Lancashire WN7 4JY
Tel: 01942 487808 www.wlct.org

Tyldesley Pool One main pool. Parent and toddler sessions Tues 10-11am and Fri 11-12pm (£1.65). Swimming lessons available from age five (10-week course £37).
Adults £2.95, Under 16s free (if you purchase a lifestyle membership card for £1.50), Under 5s free.
Castle Street, Tyldesley, Manchester M29 8EG
Tel: 01942 882722 www.wlct.org

CLASSES AND ACTIVITIES

Libraries

Most libraries in Greater Manchester provide a drop-in story or rhyme time for children under five years old. They are usually run during school term time only and are free. Some also have toy libraries and offer craft sessions and singalongs.

Libraries in Greater Manchester

Library cards can be issued from birth, with no charges being levied for late return of under fives children's books.

My children love the library and we often pop in when we are visiting the local shops. Apart from the regular story time we've also been to other free events for under fives.

Listed below are libraries in Greater Manchester and their current story time or rhyme time if confirmed.

BOLTON

Astley Bridge Moss Bank Way BL1 8NP Tel: 01204 332350 One Tues of the month 10.30am.
Blackrod Church St BL6 5EQ Tel: 01204 332380 Thurs 10.30am.
Breightmet Breightmet Drive BL2 6EE Tel: 01204 332352 One Fri of the month 11am.
Bromley Cross Toppings Estate BL7 9JL Tel: 01204 332354 Thurs 2pm.
Castle Hill Castleton Street BL2 2JW Tel: 01204 332365 One Fri of the month 9.30am.
Central Children's Le Mans Crescent BL1 1SE Tel: 01204 332180 One Thurs of the month 11am.
Farnworth Market St BL4 7PG Tel: 01204 332344 One Thurs of the month 10am.
Harwood Gate Fold BL2 3HN Tel: 01204 332340 One Fri of the month 2.30pm.
Heaton New Hall Lane BL1 5LF Tel: 01204 332357 Third Mon of the month 2.30pm.
High Street High Street BL3 6SZ Tel: 01204 332358 One Mon of the month 11am.
Horwich Jones Street BL6 7AJ Tel: 01204 332347 One Monday of the month 2.30pm.
Little Lever Coronation Square BL3 1LP Tel: 01204 332360 One Friday of the month 10am.
Marsh Lane Marsh Lane BL4 0AP

Tel: 01204 332363 One Monday of the month.
Oxford Grove Shepherd Cross Street BL1 3EJ Tel: 01204 332367 One Friday of the month 10.30am.
Westhoughton Library Street BL5 3AU Tel 01942 634640 One Friday of the month 10am.

BURY

Bury Central Manchester Road, BL9 0DG Tel: 0161 253 5871 Weds 10.30am.
Prestwich Longfield Centre M25 1AY Tel: 0161 253 7214 Thurs 10.45am.
Radcliffe Stand Lane M26 1NW Tel: 0161 253 5885 Mon 10am.
Ramsbottom Carr St BL0 9AE Tel: 0161 253 5352 Tues 2pm.
Sedgeley Park Community Room, St Gabriel's Church, Bishops Road Mon am.
Tottington Town Hall, Market Street BL8 3LN Fri 10.30am.
Unsworth Lindale Avenue, Bury BL9 8ED Tel: 0161 253 7560 Monthly Sat 11.30am.
Whitefield Pinfold Lane M45 7NY Tel: 0161 253 5548 Tues 10.15am.

MANCHESTER

Burnage Burnage Lane M19 1EW Tel: 0161 442 9036 Thurs 2.15pm.
Central St Peter's Square M2 5PD Tel: 0161 234 1900 Mon 1.30pm.
Chorlton Manchester Road M21 9PN Tel: 0161 881 3179 Thurs 10am.
Clayton Wells Centre, 101 North Road M11 4NE Tel: 0161 219 6097 Weds 9.30am.
Crumpsall Abraham Moss Centre M8 5UF Tel: 0161 908 1900 Tues 10.30am.
Didsbury 692 Wilmslow Road M20 2DN Tel: 0161 445 3220 Mon 2pm.
East City Whitworth House, Ashton Old Road M11 2WH Tel: 0161 234 5501 Thurs 2pm.
Fallowfield Platt Lane M14 7FB Tel: 0161 224 4153 Thurs 11am.
Forum The Forum, Forum Square, Wythenshawe M22 5RX Tel: 0161 935 4040 Tues 11am.
Gorton Garrett Way M18 8HE Tel: 0161 223 0775 Thurs 10am.

Higher Blackley Victoria Avenue M9 0RA Tel: 0161 740 1534 Thurs 2pm.
Hulme Stretford Road M15 5FQ Tel: 0161 226 1005 Mon 10.30am.
Longsight 519 Stockport Road M12 4NE Tel: 0161 224 1411 Mon/Weds 10.30am.
Miles Platting Varley Street M40 8EE Tel: 0161 254 7021 Second Tues of the month 10am.
New Moston Nuthurst Road M40 3PJ Tel: 0161 219 6461 Weds 10am.
North City Rochdale Road, Harpurhey M9 4AF Tel: 0161 219 6442 Thurs 10.30am.
Northenden Church Road M22 4WL Tel: 0161 998 3023 Fri 10.30am.
Rack House Yarmouth Drive M23 0BT Tel: 0161 998 2043 Weds 2.30pm.
Withington 410 Wilmslow Road M20 3BN Tel: 0161 227 3720 Weds 10.30am.

OLDHAM

For those sessions which are stated to be periodic, it is best to call ahead.
Broadway Whitegate Lane OL9 8LS Tel: 0161 624 7866 Fri 10.30am.
Chadderton Middleton Road OL9 6JN Tel: 0161 665 2225 (Periodic) Thurs 2-2.20pm, Sat 10.30-11am.
Crompton Farrow Street East, Shaw OL2 8QY Tel: 01706 842184 Toddlers Storytime and Colouring Sessions Fri 9.30am.
Failsworth Main Street M35 9DP Tel: 0161 681 2405 (Periodic) Fri 2pm.
Fitton Hill Fir Tree Avenue OL8 2QP Tel: 0161 633 2011 Mon 10.30am.
Greenfield Chew Vale OL3 7EQ Tel: 01457 872472 (Periodic) Sat 10.30am.
Limehurst Dechads Centre, Lime Green Parade OL8 3HH Tel: 0161 624 0351 Rhymetime Mon 2pm.
Oldham Cultural Quarter, Greaves Street OL1 1AL Tel: 0161 770 8000 (Periodic) Rhymetime and Tiny Tot Time.
Royton Rochdale Road OL2 6QJ Tel: 0161 770 3087 (Periodic sessions).
Uppermill St Chad's, High Street OL3 6AP Tel: 01457 872777 (Periodic) Rhymetime and Tots Time Thurs 2pm.

ROCHDALE

Alkrington Kirkway Middleton M24 1LW Tel: 0161 643 7799 Fri 11.30am.
Balderstone Balderstone Park OL11 2HD Tel: 01706 640438 Thurs 2pm.
Belfield Samson Street OL16 2XW Tel: 01706 341364 Mon 3.45pm.

Libraries

Castleton Castleton Community Centre Manchester Road OL11 3AF Tel: 01706 633430 Thurs 2pm.
Darnhill Argyle Parade Heywood OL10 3RY Tel: 01706 368142 Mon 10.30am and Thurs 10.30am. Check as may be closing in 2009 for refurbishment.
Heywood Church Street OL10 1LL Tel: 0845 2729260 Tues 2.30pm.
Junction Grimshaw Lane Middleton M24 2BW Tel: 0161 654 8910 Thurs 1.30pm.
Langley Windermere Road, Middleton M24 4LA Tel: 0161 654 8911 Fri 2pm.
Littleborough Hare Hill Park OL15 9HE Tel: 01706 378219 Tues 10.30am/ Fri 2.30pm.
Middleton Long Street Tel: 0161 643 5228 Mon 2pm.
Milnrow Newhey Road OL16 3PS Tel: 01706 641563 Fri 10am.
Norden Norden Community School Shawfield Lane OL12 7RQ Tel: 01706 631544 Thurs 1.15pm.
Smallbridge Stevenson Square, Rochdale OL12 9SA Tel: 01706 659978 Fri 10.30am.
Smithybridge 121-123 Smithybridge Road, Littleborough OL15 0BQ Tel: 01706 37828 Mon 2.30pm.
Spotland Ings Lane, Rochdale OL12 7AL Tel: 01706 648505 Tues 10.30am.
Wardle 448 Birch Road OL12 9LH Tel: 01706 377476 First/third Tues of the month 2.15pm.
Wheatsheaf Baillie Street, Rochdale OL16 1JZ Tel: 01706 924900 Mon 2.15pm. NB: Times for Rochdale story time may switch from afternoon to morning.

SALFORD

Broadwalk Broadwalk, Salford M6 5FX Tel: 0161 737 5802 Tues 10.30am.
Broughton 400-404 Bury New Rd, M7 4EY Tel: 0161 792 6640 Mon 10.30am.
Cadishead 126 Liverpool Rd M44 5AN Tel: 0161 775 3457 Mon 9.30am and 11.15am.
Clifton Community Centre, 6 Wynne Ave M27 8FU Tel: 0161 794 1591 Weds 2pm.
Eccles Gateway, 28 Barton Lane M30 0TU Tel: 0161 909 6528 Thurs 2pm.
Height King Street, Salford M6 7GY Tel: 0161 736 1907 Tues 2pm.
Irlam Hurst Fold, Liverpool Road M44 6FD Tel: 0161 775 3566 Thurs 9.30am and 11.15am.
Little Hulton Longshaw Drive M28 0AZ Tel: 0161 790 4201 Tues 11am, Weds 1.30pm, Thurs 9.30am and 11am.

Ordsall Ordsall Neighbourhood Office, Robert Hall Street M5 3LT Tel: 0161 603 4097 Tues 11am.
Swinton Chorley Road M27 4AE. Tel: 0161 921 2370 Tues 11am, Thurs 11am and 2pm.
Walkden Gateway, 2 Smith Street M28 3EZ Tel: 0161 909 6518 Tues 11am.
Winton Old Parrin Lane M30 8BY Tel: 0161 921 2180, Tues 9.30am and 11am.

STOCKPORT

Bramhall Bramhall Lane South SK7 2DU Tel: 0845 6444307 Tues 2pm.
Bredbury George Lane SK6 1DJ Tel: 0845 6444307 Tues 2pm.
Brinnington 367 Brinnington Road Tel: 0845 6444307 Mon 2pm.
Cheadle Ashfield Road,SK8 1BB Tel: 08456 444307 Thurs 2pm.
Cheadle Hulme Mellor Road SK8 5AU Tel: 0845 6444307 Tues 2pm.
Dialstone Lisburne Lane, Offerton SK2 7LL Tel: 0845 6444307 Mon 11am.
Edgeley Edgeley Road, Stockport SK3 9NB Tel: 0845 6444307 Mon 2pm.
Great Moor Gladstone Street SK2 7QF Tel: 0845 6444307 Weds 2pm.
Hazel Grove Beech Avenue SK7 4QP Tel: 0845 6444307 Tues 11am.
Heald Green Finney Green SK8 3JB Tel: 0845 6444307 Sat 11am.
Heatons Thornfield Road, Heaton Moor SK4 3LD Tel: 0845 6444307 Mon 2.15pm.
High Lane Buxton Road SK6 8DX Tel: 0845 6444307 Mon 2.30pm.
Marple Memorial Park SK6 6BA Tel: 0845 6444307 Tues 2pm.
Reddish Gorton Road SK5 6UG Tel: 0845 6444307 Fri 2pm.

TAMESIDE

Droylsden Manchester Road M43 6EP Tel: 0161 370 1282 Mon 9.30am.
Denton Peel Street M34 3JY Tel: 0161 336 8234 Thurs 2.15pm.
Hattersley Hattersley Road East SK14 3EQ Tel: 0161 368 8515 Mon 2pm.
Haughton Green Mancunian Road, Denton M34 7NP Tel: 0161 336 7193 Mon 2.15pm.
Mottram Broadbottom Road SK14 6JA Tel: 01457 764144 Mon 1.15pm.
Newton Talbot Road, Hyde SK14 4HH Tel: 0161 366 0290 Tues 1.30pm.
Stalybridge Trinity Street SK15 2BN Tel: 0161 338 3831 Tues 9.30am.
Tameside Central Old Street OL6 7SG Tel: 0161 342 2030 Tues 2pm.

TRAFFORD

Altrincham 20 Stamford New Rd WA14 1EJ Tel: 0161 912 5920 Tues/Thurs 11am.
Coppice Coppice Avenue Sale M33 4ND Tel: 0161 912 3560 Tues 2.15pm.
Davyhulme Hayeswater Road M41 7BL Tel: 0161 912 2880 Mon 10.30am.
Greatstone Stretford Leisure Centre, Greatstone Road M32 0ZS Tel: 0161 912 4815 Weds 10am.
Hale Leigh Road WA15 9BG Tel: 0161 912 5966 Tues 2pm.
Lostock Selby Road, Stretford M32 9PL Tel:0161 912 5226 Mon 2pm.
Partington Central Road M31 4EL Tel: 0161 912 5450 Thurs 10.15am.
Sale Waterside M33 7ZF Tel: 0161 912 3008 Tues 2.15pm.
Stretford Kingsway M32 8AP Tel: 0161 912 5150 Tues 2.15pm.
Timperley 405 Stockport Road WA15 7XR Tel: 0161 912 5600 Mon 2.30pm.
Urmston 38-42 Moorfield Walk M41 0TT Tel: 0161 912 2727 Weds 2.30pm.
Woodsend Woodsend Road, Flixton M41 8GN Tel: 0161 912 2919 Thurs 2pm.

WIGAN

Ashton Wigan Road WN4 9BH Tel: 01942 727119 Weds 10.30am and 2pm, Sun 11.00am.
Aspull Oakfield Crescent WN2 1XJ Tel:01942 831303 Tues 10am.
Atherton York Street M46 9JH Tel:01942 404817 Weds 10am.
Beech Hill Buckley Street West WN6 7PQ Tel: 01942 747750 Weds 2pm.
Golborne Tanners Lane, Warrington WA3 3AW Tel: 01942 777800 Fri 2pm.
Hindley Market Street WN2 3AN Tel: 01942 255287 Tues 10.30am.
Ince Smithy Green WN2 2AT Tel: 01942 324423 Tues 2pm.
Leigh Turnpike Centre, Civic Square, Market St WN7 1EB Tel: 01942 404404 Weds 11am and 1.30pm.
Marsh Green Harrow Road WN5 0QL Tel: 01942 760041 Tues 2pm.
Ornell Ornell Post WN5 8LY Tel: 01942 705060 Thurs 1.45pm.
Platt Bridge Platt Bridge Community First, Rivington Avenue WN2 5NG Tel: 01942 487997 Thurs 11am.
Shelvington Gathurst Lane WN6 8HA Tel: 01257 252618 Weds 10.30am.
Standish Cross St WN6 0HQ Tel: 01257 400496 Tues 2pm.
Tyldesley Stanley St M29 8AH Tel: 01942 404738 Mon 2pm.
Wiend Children's Centre, Millgate, Wigan WN1 1PF Weds 2pm.

Shopping

The range of shops in Greater Manchester is extensive and you need go nowhere else. With a baby in tow it's useful to know where you can change a nappy or breastfeed in private.

Shopping

MANCHESTER CITY CENTRE

Boots Stocks everything from prams to medicines, toys and clothes all suitable for under 5s. There is a baby room on the first floor adjacent to the baby department which includes a breastfeeding room, changing facilities and a bottle warmer. There are no customer toilets though.
Boots, 32 Market Street, Manchester M1 1PL
Tel: 0161 832 6533 www.boots.com

House of Fraser (Kendals) Kendals is a good "one-stop shop" kind of place. Parking is on site – though this is pricey and I find the double doors from the car park into the store a complete nightmare! There's a very child friendly restaurant (see café section on page 62) and the children's clothing department with Hamleys toy shop situated on the 6th floor are lovely. There is lift access. Baby changing is on the 3rd and 6th floor – the latter of these has three steps up to them.
House of Fraser, Deansgate, Manchester M60 3AU
Tel; 0161 832 3414 www.houseoffraser.co.uk

Manchester Arndale Centre contains a lot of eateries, which are easy to navigate with pushchairs plus an interesting food market. Check out the excellent fish stall. There's plenty of baby changing, nursing chairs and parent and toddler toilets. Bottle warming facilities can be found in the Foodchain.
Manchester Arndale, Manchester M4 3AQ
Tel: 0161 833 9851   www.manchesterarndale.com

Waterstones On the second floor of this centrally located book shop there are baby-changing facilities next to Costa Coffee. Costa will also supply hot water for heating up baby food and they have high chairs. Lift access.
Waterstones, 91 Deansgate, Manchester M3 2BW
Tel: 0161 837 3000   www.waterstones.com

MANCHESTER FORT

Just a few minutes drive out of the city centre at Manchester Fort is a selection of purpose built shops along with free parking.
Mamas & Papas You'll probably already be familiar with this brand's products from when you were getting ready to have your baby, but M&P is worth re-visiting as it has a very good children's clothing range, well-designed educational toys with great walkers and push-alongs. They also offer a really useful car-seat fitting service. There is a demonstration area where trained staff will show you how to fit their car seats. Where possible, they will also take the seat out to your car to ensure it fits correctly and securely.
Mamas & Papas, Manchester Fort Shopping Park, Cheetham Hill Road, Manchester M8 8EP
Tel: 0845 268 2000 www.mamasandpapas.co.uk

Borders A large book store with a fabulous children's department. Children and toddlers are encouraged to sit on the brightly coloured floor and stools and enjoy the books. Weekly activities are held to encourage reading and there's an in-store Starbucks where you can grab a coffee. Baby change facilities are available.
Borders, Manchester Fort Shopping Park, Cheetham Hill Road, Manchester M8 8EP
Tel: 0161 833 0208 www.bordersstores.co.uk

JOHN LEWIS

John Lewis at Cheadle is fairly unbeatable in terms of child-friendliness. The baby changing facilities are always spotlessly clean, there are free nappy and wipe dispensers, bottle warming facilities and nursing chairs. The café welcomes mums and tots and the staff will help you to your table with trays and provide bottle warmers. There are children's meals available for those with toddlers or a free baby jar with an adults meal. John Lewis will also loan you a pushchair if you've forgotten yours.
John Lewis, Wilmslow Road, Cheadle, Cheshire SK8 3BZ Tel: 0161 491 4914 www.johnlewis.com

THE TRAFFORD CENTRE

I think I've finally mastered the art of being able to shop and keep a toddler entertained at the same time… The Trafford Centre holds the key!

For £2.50 an hour, you can hire a Little Tikes Car Buggy – one of those they sit in and "steer" and you push them round (You need to leave a £20 deposit).

There are also various distractions if toddlers start getting a bit fractious. Near John Lewis you'll find the 'Jumping Fountain' – which shoots huge jets of water 50ft in the air. You'll also find face painting on the second level near The Orient restaurant area – £3.50 per face for a rather good little tiger or butterfly following you round.

Every day at 1pm and 3pm you can take the children to see Barney Bear – a large teddy bear driving a red car. He can be found by the statues in New Orleans in the restaurant area.

The tour de force though is the Crèche and Play Area situated in The Orient on the ground floor. The Play area (suitable for 0-10 year olds) includes two ball pools, two wavy slides, climbing nets, tube

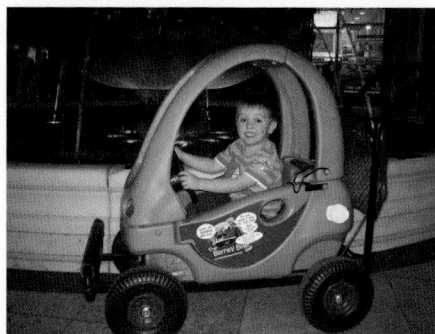

Having fun in the little cars at The Trafford Centre.

crawls and rope swings. For children under six there is a dedicated Little Tikes Play area. It costs £2.10 for half hour play. Security measures are reassuringly rigorous.

There's a children's drinking fountain, toilets, baby changing and baby feeding room all within the area, plus a vending machine for nappies.

The Crèche is available for children aged from two to eight years old. Again there's an adventure play structure, Little Tikes toys, Sega and Play Station games, play dough, sand play and a home corner. Prices start from £2 per half hour (this rate not available at weekends and holidays) to £7.90 for two and a half hours, the maximum stay.

Security wristbands (free) and pushchairs for you to borrow (ID and a £20 cash deposit) are available from Customer Services in the main dome.

All of the Trafford Centre toilet areas include parent and child toilets and unisex baby changing facilities (no supplies, but vending machines selling nappies) and a breast feeding room.

The following shops also have excellent facilities: **Boots** has a dedicated baby room at the back of the shop on the ground floor. You'll find bottle warming machines, baby changing stations, nursing chairs and a children's toilet.

John Lewis has a dedicated parent room near the toy area on the ground floor. You'll find a bottle warmer, screened areas for baby feeding, changing stations, a nappy dispenser (£1.50 each), a drinking fountain and a parent and child toilet. In their restaurant, John Lewis offers a free jar of organic baby food with an adult meal purchased (they do not heat up your own baby food or bottles).

Debenhams Outside the entrance on the ground floor you'll find unisex baby changing (plus a vending machine with nappy and wipes for £1.50) a parent and child toilet and a nursing room. On the first floor, there are more changing facilities in the toilets next to the bedding dept. The spacious Style Café also on the first floor has a baby food and bottle warming station

INDEPENDENT TOY SHOPS

Rumpus, Didsbury A pleasure to shop in – manager Louise is always ready to help steer you in the direction of the perfect present. Specialises in toys for children aged 0-8 years. Plenty of toys around for the children to play with whilst you look round. Recently included in the Guardian's list of top independent retailers.
Rumpus, 2 Albert Hill Street, Didsbury, Manchester M20 6RF Tel: 0161 445 1097 www.rumpustoys.co.uk

Toys & Tales, Bramhall A fairly large shop stocking toys from birth and brands such as Playmobil, Sylvanian Families, Thomas and Steiff. There's a great collection of dressing up clothes, books, jigsaws and musical instruments (including a very good range of guitars). There's a sofa in one area with toy tables for the children to play at. Plus beautiful art canvas' and prints for children painted by owner Kaye.
Toys & Tales, 44-46 Bramhall Lane South, Bramhall, Stockport, Cheshire SK7 1AH
Tel: 0161 439 6002 www.toysandtales.com

Toto's, Altrincham Children's clothes shop that has large range of toys as well including Steiff bears, Playmobil, Sylvannian Families and Galt
Toto's, 5 Grafton Street, Altrincham, WA14 1DH
Tel: 0161 928 7657 www.totos.co.uk

Little Nut Tree Toys, Chorlton Stocks more unique and unusual brands of toys sourced mainly from Europe. The shelves are crammed with puppets, (very affordable) wooden train sets & accessories that are compatible with the big brands, marble runs, a good selection of "pocket money" toys, learning aids and sticker books.
Little Nut Tree Toys, 93 Manchester Road, Chorlton, Manchester M21 9GA
Tel: 0844 800 8574 www.littlenuttreetoys.co.uk

Oklahoma, Northern Quarter, Manchester Primarily a gift shop aimed at adults, there are also lots for little ones including wind-up donkeys, kitsch lunch boxes, Whoopee cushions and Fisher Price retro toys.
Oklahoma, 74-76 High Street, Manchester M4 1ES
Tel: 0161 834 1136

Little Treasures, Ramsbottom As well as a great range in toys, Little Treasures specialises in beautiful bespoke children's furniture made by owner Jamie, member of the Guild of Master Craftsmen.
Little Treasures, 47 Bolton Street, Ramsbottom, Lancashire BL0 9HU
Tel: 01706 828644 www.yourlittletreasures.co.uk

Traditional Toys, Bolton Specialising in timeless wooden toys, such as rocking horses, Italian hand-made rag dolls, the Paddington Bear collection, Beatrix Potter products, wooden dolls houses, trikes and trailors.
Traditional Toys, The Last Drop Village, Bolton BL7 9PZ
Tel: 01204 597862 www.traditionaltoyshop.co.uk

Fun Time Toys, Leigh Stock mostly pre-school toys with big brands such as Leapfrog, Tomy, V-tech, Character Options and Wow. Also sell nursery equipment.
Fun Time Toys, 108 Bradshawgate, Leigh WN7 4NP
Tel: 01942 608300

Shopping

(including a microwave). They sell Cow & Gate baby jars, starting at 95p and there's children's deli-boxes or hot meals available for £3.35 with free crayons and fun sheets. A kids' three-item breakfast for £2.15 is served until 11.30am.

Selfridges Next to Paperchase on Selfridge's first floor, there are two baby changing rooms.
Trafford Centre Mon-Fri 10am-10pm, Sat 10am-8pm, Sun 12noon-6pm.
The Trafford Centre, Jn 9 or 10 off the M60, Manchester M17 8AA
Tel: 0161 749 1510 www.traffordcentre.co.uk
Creche & Play area Tel: 0161 746 9000
Shuttle bus connecting the centre to the Metrolink at Stretford.

BENTS

Bents offers so much more than just gardening supplies and plants which is what it set out to sell originally. There is a wonderful food emporium selling organic ranges for babies and children, a toy department and a children's clothing and baby section.

The Fresh Approach restaurant has a large array of open sandwiches, cakes and treats and if you've forgotten to pack baby's lunch then a free jar of baby food is offered with an adult meal. The restaurant is self-service and the staff are happy to carry your tray to your table if you have a pram or just need a hand. Highchairs are available along with baby changing facilities.

If you are only going to make one trip to Bents with young children then I would recommend doing so during the Christmas season, even if you don't celebrate Christmas. Santa's tea parties and breakfasts are held for children aged from three years from the end of November until Christmas but they have to be booked in advance.

Winners of Cheshire's Best Tourism Retail Attraction and Best Garden Centre in the North West 2008.
Mon-Fri 8.30am-9pm, Sat 8.30am-5.30pm, Sun 9am-5pm
Bents, Warrington Road, Glazebury, Warrington, Cheshire WA3 5NT Tel: 01942 266300 www.bents.co.uk

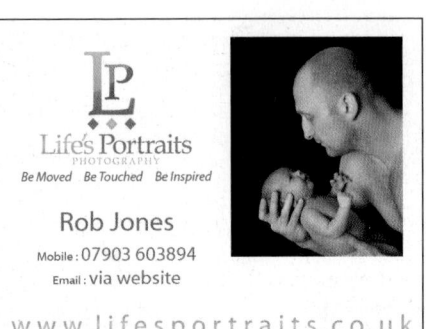
So, having provided you with lots of things to do with your babies and toddlers, we felt it only right to offer some activities for mum. Whilst most are essential and educative, mums should enjoy the high life every now and again.

Mum's Directory

Buggyfit is a fun, energising outdoor exercise class designed specifically for new mums, they're an hour long and usually involve a 3-5 mile route. Classes start with a moderate warm up walk, moving into a power walk or run along with exercises to strengthen and tone specific muscles.
Sessions cost from £4.50 and classes held in Chorlton, Didsbury, Appleton, Northwich, Altrincham and Rochdale. Tel: 0771 318 3522 www.buggyfit.co.uk

Cottontails Nappy Laundry Service deliver freshly laundered pure cotton nappies to your door on the same day each week at the same time collecting the soiled nappies for laundering. Several local authorities allow you to try the nappy laundry service free of charge for a trial month, contact Cottontails direct to see if you qualify.
Greater Manchester, Cheshire and Lancashire. Cost is £9.25 per week/£40 per month.
Tel: 01244 374521 www.cottontails.co.uk

Greater Manchester Fire Service offer a free home fire risk assessment service that everyone should take up. You simply book an appointment and a week later three firemen arrive along with a fire engine to your house, you can just imagine my little boy's face! After a few questions, the crew then inspect your house and install brand new (free) smoke alarms wherever necessary. They also advise you on an escape plan in case of a fire. It is important that children know what they should do and it is a good idea for them to hear the alarm when you test it. The assessment takes less than half an hour and is an excellent service offered throughout Greater Manchester.
Tel: 0800 555 815 www.manchesterfire.gov.uk

Glo Family offer a brilliant and unique range of Childbirth Preparation Courses and Pre/Postnatal Fitness Classes in Manchester & Cheshire. Glo Family's Antenatal courses which run over two weekends, give couples the opportunity to prepare fully for labour and birth. New for 2009 are some great courses for all mums, including Fit Mums Bikini Bootcamp, a 45 minute exercise and weight loss program. Each week you will be weighed and measured and receive tips and advice on positive eating, A course is two sessions a week for six weeks costing £75. Glo Family will also be running Group Postnatal Personal Training and Mums on Mats – a fitness pilates class. Babies in car seats are welcome at both.
Tel: 0844 800 7380 www.glofamily.com

The Happy Mum is a self improvement coaching service – just for mums. The aim is to boost your confidence, help

you feel motivated, raise your self-esteem and maximise your potential.
Tel: 0161 777 6744 www.thehappymum.co.uk

Heaven Spa based at the Hilton hotel in Beetham Tower, central Manchester and in Didsbury, they offer special packages for pre and post-natal luxury pampering. You can enjoy Mello Mama, Lighten Up and The Yummy Tummy. Once you've had your baby and are in need of a special treat, try the 4th Trimester Healing Hour – a relaxing top to toe massage to help realign and restore your body for £60, money well spent!
*Heaven Spa, 115 Lapwing Lane, Didsbury M20 6UR
Tel: 0161 448 8786
Heaven Spa, 2nd Floor, Hilton Manchester, Deansgate M3 4LQ
Tel: 0161 870 1789 www.heaven-spa.co.uk*

The National Childbirth Trust provides expert information and trusted practical and emotional support through a fantastic network of groups run by volunteer mums and dads. Each local branch has a busy social calendar for parents with babies of all ages; from days out with other families to Bumps and Babies Groups, Cheeky Monkeys Tea Parties and Nearly New Sales. The NCT also has a pregnancy and birth and a breastfeeding helpline which you do not need to be a member to call.
*Pregnancy & Birth Tel: 0870 4448709 Mon-Sun 8am-10pm
Breastfeeding Line Tel: 0300 330 0771 Mon-Thurs
9am-5pm, Fri 9am-4pm
Enquiries Tel: 0300 33 00 770 www.nct.org.uk.*

Pushy Mothers offers an effective, safe and specific one-hour workout with no childcare concerns as you bring baby along whatever the weather. With lots of cardio pushing, it burns baby fat, tightens and tones muscles, flattens tummy and keeps you yummy! Classes cost £5 per session and are booked in blocks of four. There is a one-off membership fee of £15 and you will receive a Pushy Mothers bag with gifts plus discount vouchers. Classes in Didsbury
Tel: 07730 765 954 www.pushymothers.com

St Johns Ambulance hold a specific child and infant Emergency Life Support Course. Designed to teach you how to deal with an emergency and CPR skills specific to children and infants, it is ideal for parents, grandparents or guardians. The course covers, amongst other things, managing an incident, child and infant resuscitation, treatment of severe bleeding, unconsciousness and choking in children and infants. Courses cost £18 plus vat and tend to run on a Saturday (three hours) out of Stockport and Oldham. Definitely put this course on your 'to do' list.
St John House, Crossley Road, Heaton Chapel, Stockport SK4 5BF Tel: 08714 236030 www.sja.org.uk

SureStart is based in children's centres throughout Manchester. Families can source local information and have access to free services including early education and childcare, advice on parenting, local childcare options, health screening, health visitor services, breast-feeding support and helping parents back into work. For your nearest SureStart centre please check their website or call.
Tel: 0870 000 2288 www.surestart.gov.uk

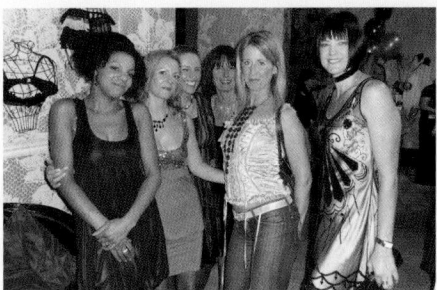
Mums at an Inner Glo event at Agent Provocateur.

Unicorn Grocery is a vegan superstore located in Chorlton, brilliant for seasonal organic fruit and vegetables, ideal for when you start weaning and pureeing. Everything's ethically sourced so you buy with a clear conscience. The baby selection is first rate – they sell the Earth Friendly baby care range, alongside cloth nappies, biodegradable wipes, organic baby grows and they have a good selection of fruit purees. For those shopping with toddlers there's a cute little play area kitted out with a wooden kitchen, puzzles and giant blackboard. Unicorn Grocery is a workers co-operative which is competitively priced and well worth supporting to try and stem the ever-tightening grip of the huge multi-nationals. Unicorn won *Radio 4's* Best Local Food Retailer Award 2008.
Unicorn Grocery, 89 Albany Road, Chorlton, Manchester M21 0BN Tel: 0161 861 0010 www.unicorn-grocery.co.uk

And finally...

Inner Glo is time to relax and have fun. It's a wonderfully glamorous social networking group for mums in Manchester and Cheshire. Members have the opportunity to attend monthly social events, which can range from a private fashion show at Selfridges; an extravagant Bollywood night at a top Indian restaurant or even burlesque dancing lessons! Champagne is always served and fantastic goodie bags are handed out at the end of the evening. The concept is about doing something for yourself; whether it's making useful contacts for your business, learning a new skill or simply having a fun night out. So, put the kids to bed, slip on a pair of heels and go do something just for you...
*Annual Cost: Silver Membership £30, Gold Membership £95
www.innerglo.co.uk*

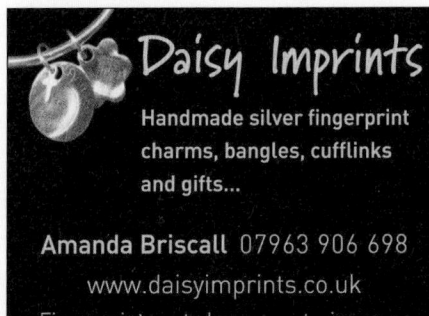

USEFUL INFORMATION

Getting around

Greater Manchester has one of the friendliest public transport networks in the country. What could be nicer than riding on a bus, train or tram where you can spend some quality time with your little one? However, if you're daunted by taking young children on buses, trains or trams then hopefully this section provided by GMPTE will give you some reassurance beforehand that you will manage your child, buggy and all the other bits and bobs you need.

Travelling in and around Greater Manchester

On weekdays we recommend that you start your journey after the morning rush hour – after 9.30am – when services are less busy and there is more space to carry a pushchair. Train and Metrolink tram tickets cost less at 'off-peak' times which are after 9.30am on weekdays and all day on Saturday, Sunday and public holidays. Children under five travel free and if you're over 60 and taking the grandchildren on a day trip, it doesn't get cheaper than this.

Buses

Buses are particularly handy because there's probably a route and a stop near where you live. Modern buses are child-friendly with wide doors and space to store your buggy. If the bus is busy you might need to fold your buggy.

On newer buses, the driver can lower their bus to pavement level to let you get on and off easily. Accessible buses are shown in bus timetables with a wheelchair symbol.

When you arrive in Manchester city centre there are two main bus stations – at Piccadilly Gardens and Shudehill Interchange. Buses leaving these stations connect to other towns, suburbs and countryside of Greater Manchester. There are also plenty of bus stops convenient for other parts of the city.

As well as single tickets many bus companies offer returns and day tickets that can be used on all the services run by that company – so check with the driver.

Trains

Local trains are a great way to travel with many well-located stations in Manchester and other local town centres. Trains are spacious, comfortable and most have toilets and plenty of luggage space.

There are five train stations in the centre of Manchester. Piccadilly and Victoria are main stations and Oxford Road, Deansgate and Salford Central are served by many local routes. All main stations have baby-changing facilities.

Stations vary in their design and many have ramps for your buggy. Some still have steps plus there is usually a step up onto the train. The rail map on page 90 shows the routes and the stations that have parking and step-free access.

If you don't live near a station, many have free car parking and the price of a ticket will often be less than petrol and car parking at your destination.

If you buy a rail ticket to Manchester centre from a Greater Manchester rail station (see rail map) you can use it to travel free on Metrolink trams in Manchester city centre.

All single and return train tickets cost less at off-peak times. At off-peak times you can also buy a Rail Ranger ticket that lets you to travel anywhere in Greater Manchester. An Evening Ranger ticket allows the same travel after 6.30pm. Buy your ticket from the ticket office or from the conductor on the train if this is closed.

Tip – if you already have a rail season ticket

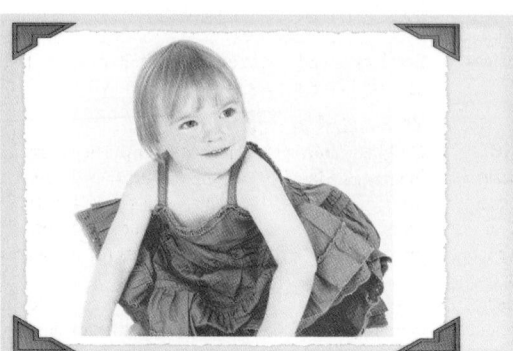

USEFUL INFORMATION

between two Greater Manchester rail stations you can use it to travel anywhere in Greater Manchester at weekends and public holidays!
National Rail Enquiries 08457 48 49 50
www.nationalrail.co.uk

Metrolink trams

Greater Manchester's Metrolink trams provide links between Bury, Altrincham, or Salford Quays and Eccles to Manchester city centre.

Metrolink was specially designed with easy access so there is no gap between the platform edge and the tram itself and all stops have either a ramp, lift or escalator access. The central section of the tram is an area specifically designed for wheelchairs and prams. The sign on the platform (disabled access) will tell you where to wait to board at the correct doors on the vehicle. Under 5s travel free and children over five pay half fare.

A MetroMax ticket lets you make as many tram journeys as you like for a whole day and are available at any time. Buy your ticket from the

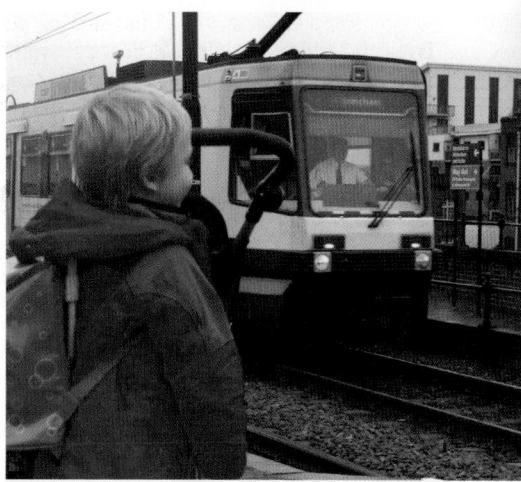

Ollie at G-Mex Metrolink station. The metro offers a link between north and south Manchester. They are a great addition to the city and children love them.

Metrolink

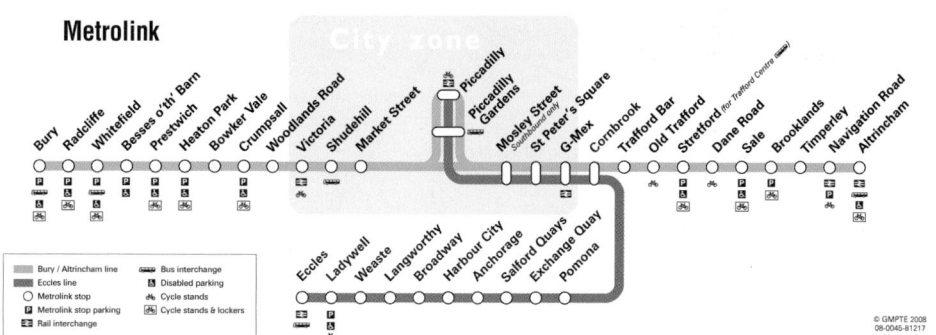

ticket machine at the Metrolink stop before you make your journey.

Trams run frequently, generally during the day every six minutes on the Bury and Altrincham lines and every 12 minutes on the Eccles line, so there isn't a timetable – simply turn up and wait for the next one.
Metrolink Customer Services 0161 205 2000
www.metrolink.co.uk

Getting around Manchester city centre

Metroshuttle is the name of the free bus services running around Manchester's city centre streets. There are three circular routes, covering all of the main city centre areas. Metroshuttle buses are low-floor, easy access with a frequency of about every five minutes on Service 1 (orange), every 10 minutes on Service 2 (green) and every 10 minutes on Service 3 (purple).

Metroshuttle links Piccadilly, Victoria, Oxford Road and Deansgate rail stations and many bus and Metrolink tram stops. So whatever the reason for your visit, you can use Metroshuttle to get around, hopping on and off as often as you wish.

All three services run Mon-Sat 7am-7pm. Services 1 and 2 run on Sundays 10am-6pm. (No service 3 on Sundays).

Your ticket to ride

Children under five travel free on public transport in Greater Manchester when they travel with adults. You can buy single or return tickets from the driver on buses, from ticket machines (before you board) on tram stops, or from ticket offices (or on board) for local trains.

If you are making a few trips or using a combination of buses, trains and trams then day tickets available.

MANCHESTER CITY CENTRE

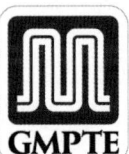

GMPTE

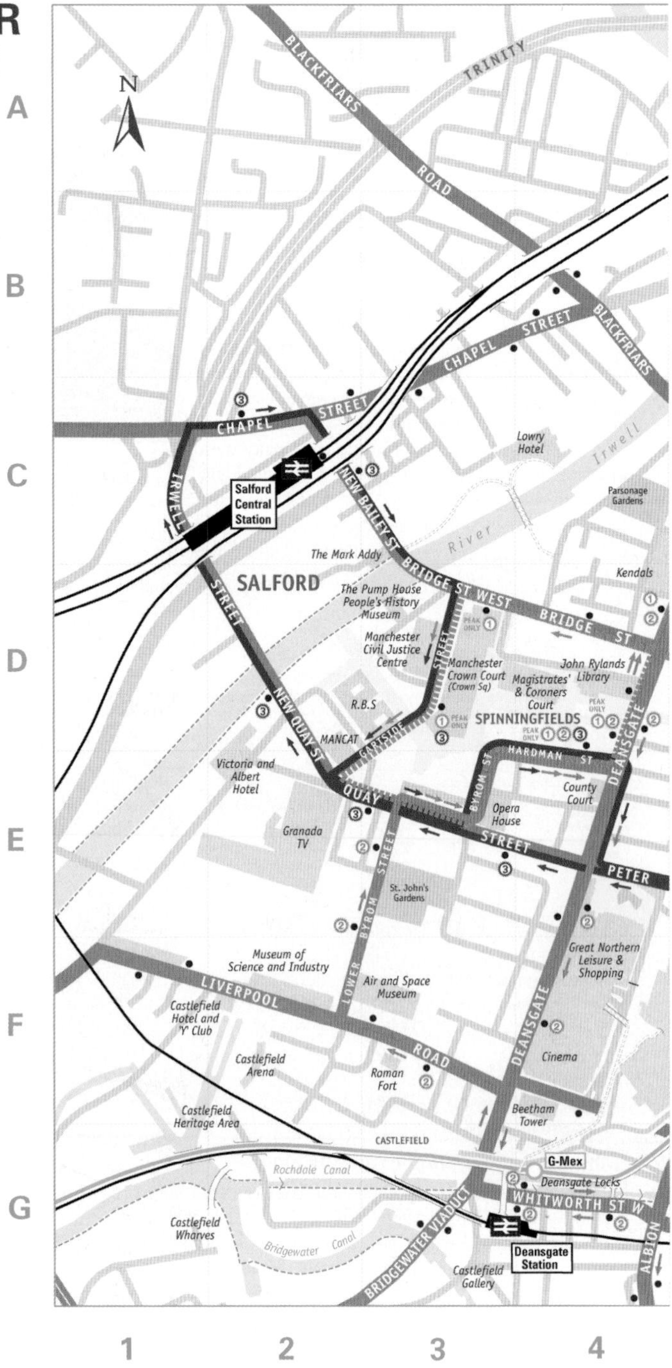

0	100	200 yards
0	100	200 metres

Legend:

- ●━━ Road with bus route/bus stop
- ▦ Road without bus route
- ▤ Motorway
- → One way street
- ➕ Train line & station
- ─○─ Metrolink tram line & stop
- ⓘ Information centre
- ═ Bridge
- Pedestrianised area or road
- Featured building
- Park or garden
- Water, lock & towpath
- Footpath

METROSHUTTLE:
Free buses linking all parts of the city centre

- ① Route 1 and bus stop
- ① Route 1 peak time only
- ② Route 2 and bus stop
- ③ Route 3 and bus stop

USEFUL INFORMATION

Map labels: Manchester City Centre map showing streets and landmarks including Blackfriars Road, Trinity, Chapel Street, Blackfriars Street, Lowry Hotel, Parsonage Gardens, Kendals, Salford Central Station, The Mark Addy, Bridge St West, Bridge St, River Irwell, Irwell Street, SALFORD, The Pump House People's History Museum, Manchester Civil Justice Centre, Manchester Crown Court (Crown Sq), Magistrates' & Coroners Court, John Rylands Library, Deansgate, New Bailey St, New Quay St, R.B.S., MANCAT, SPINNINGFIELDS, Hardman Street, Byrom St, Victoria and Albert Hotel, Granada TV, Quay Street, Opera House, County Court, Peter Street, St. John's Gardens, Museum of Science and Industry, Air and Space Museum, Lower Byrom Street, Liverpool Road, Castlefield Hotel and 'Y' Club, Castlefield Arena, Roman Fort, Great Northern Leisure & Shopping, Cinema, Deansgate, Beetham Tower, Castlefield Heritage Area, CASTLEFIELD, Rochdale Canal, G-Mex, Deansgate Locks, Whitworth St W, Castlefield Wharves, Bridgewater Viaduct, Bridgewater Canal, Deansgate Station, Castlefield Gallery, Albion.

Grid: A B C D E F G / 1 2 3 4

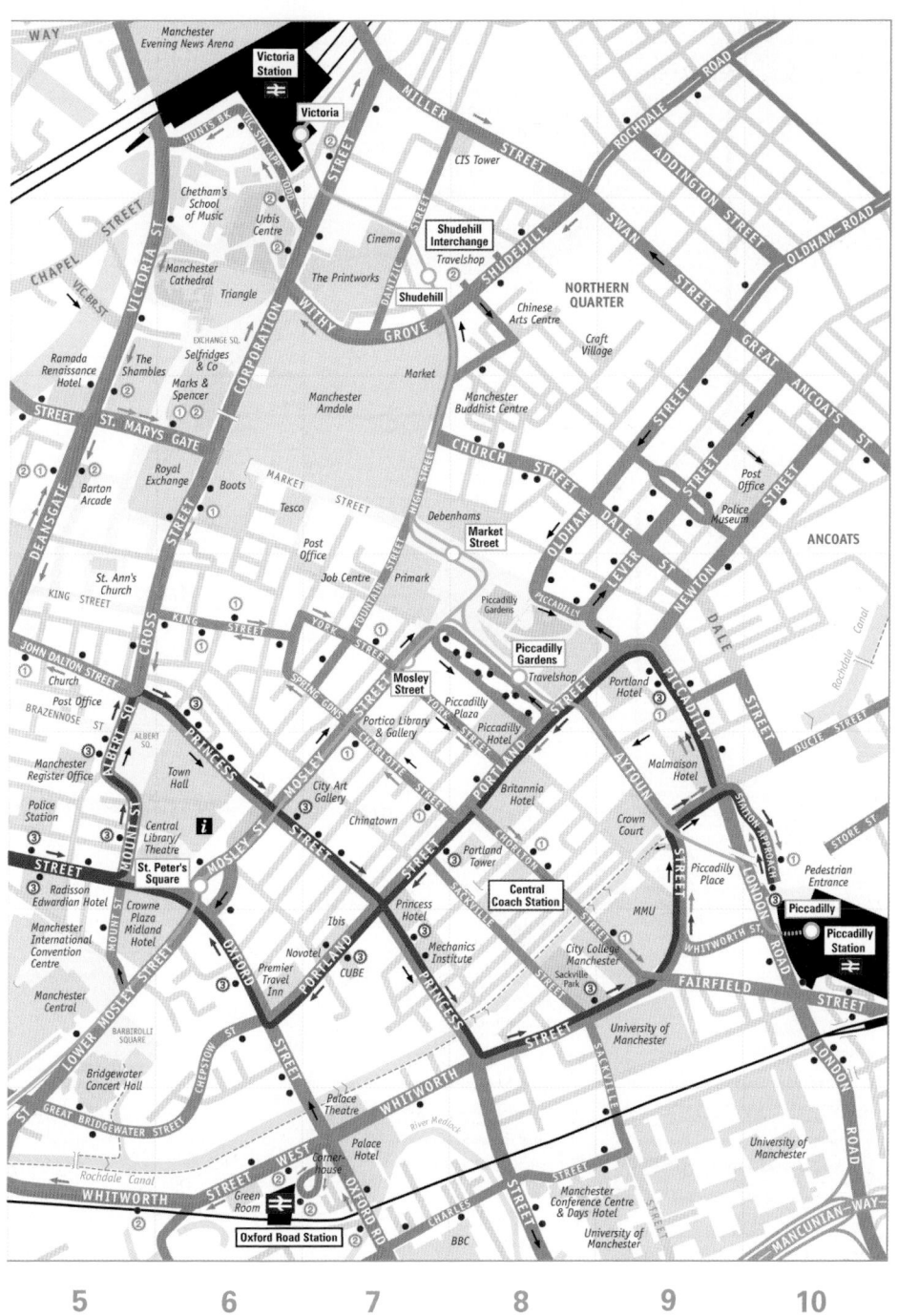

Getting around

Greater Manchester Rail Network

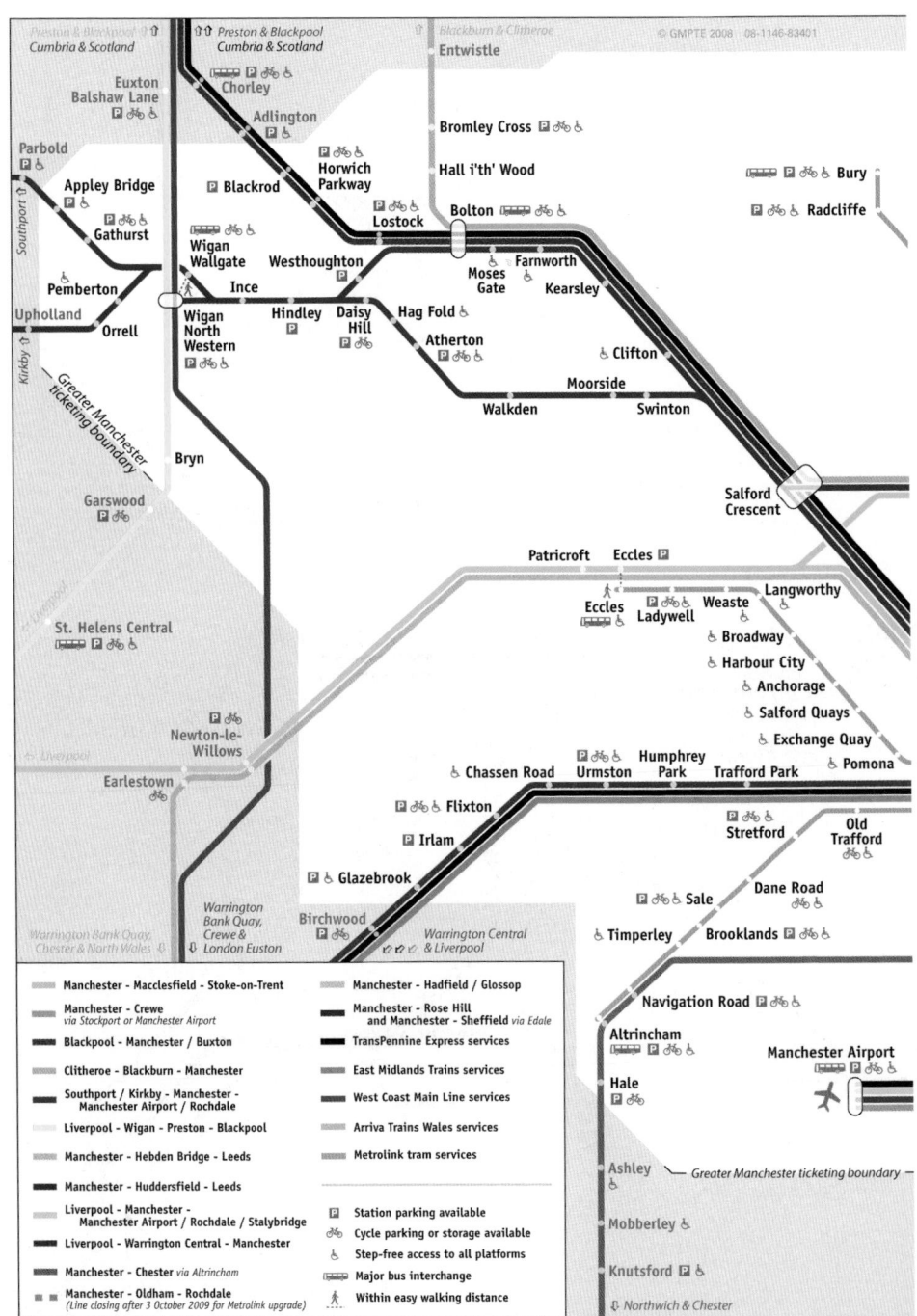

Manchester - Macclesfield - Stoke-on-Trent

Manchester - Crewe via Stockport or Manchester Airport

Blackpool - Manchester / Buxton

Clitheroe - Blackburn - Manchester

Southport / Kirkby - Manchester - Manchester Airport / Rochdale

Liverpool - Wigan - Preston - Blackpool

Manchester - Hebden Bridge - Leeds

Manchester - Huddersfield - Leeds

Liverpool - Manchester - Manchester Airport / Rochdale / Stalybridge

Liverpool - Warrington Central - Manchester

Manchester - Chester via Altrincham

Manchester - Oldham - Rochdale (Line closing after 3 October 2009 for Metrolink upgrade)

Manchester - Hadfield / Glossop

Manchester - Rose Hill and Manchester - Sheffield via Edale

TransPennine Express services

East Midlands Trains services

West Coast Main Line services

Arriva Trains Wales services

Metrolink tram services

🅿 Station parking available

🚲 Cycle parking or storage available

♿ Step-free access to all platforms

🚌 Major bus interchange

🚶 Within easy walking distance

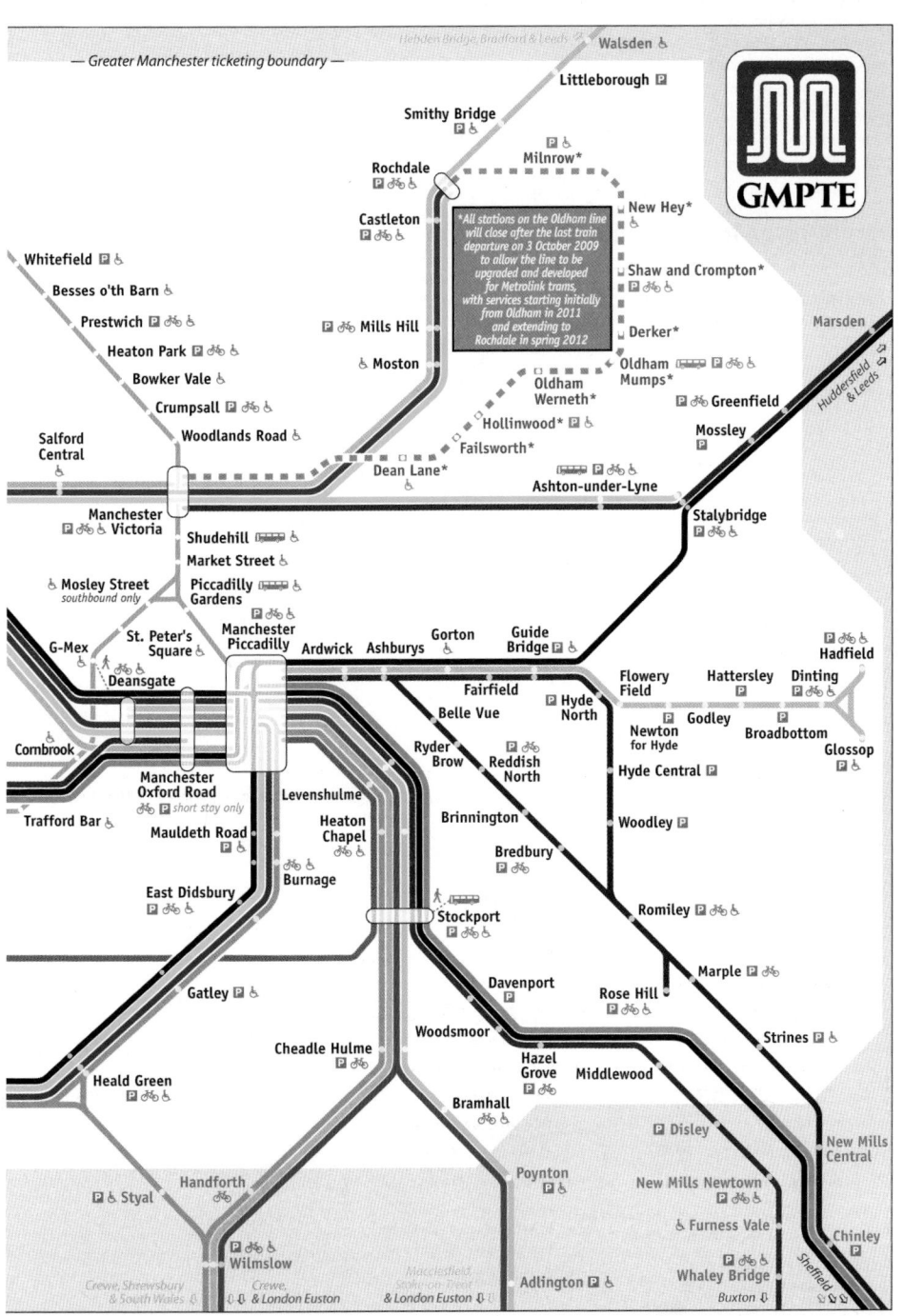

Greater Manchester ticketing boundary —

Hebden Bridge, Bradford & Leeds

Walsden

Littleborough

Smithy Bridge

Milnrow*

Rochdale

Castleton

New Hey*

*All stations on the Oldham line
will close after the last train
departure on 3 October 2009
to allow the line to be
upgraded and developed
for Metrolink trams,
with services starting initially
from Oldham in 2011
and extending to
Rochdale in spring 2012

Whitefield

Shaw and Crompton*

Besses o'th Barn

Mills Hill

Prestwich

Marsden

Heaton Park

Derker*

Bowker Vale

Moston

Oldham Mumps*

Crumpsall

Oldham Werneth*

Greenfield

Woodlands Road

Hollinwood*

Mossley

Salford Central

Failsworth*

Dean Lane*

Ashton-under-Lyne

Huddersfield & Leeds

Manchester Victoria

Shudehill

Stalybridge

Market Street

Mosley Street
southbound only

Piccadilly Gardens

St. Peter's Square

Manchester Piccadilly

Ardwick

Ashburys

Gorton

Guide Bridge

G-Mex

Deansgate

Hadfield

Fairfield

Flowery Field

Hattersley

Dinting

Combrook

Belle Vue

Hyde North

Godley

Newton for Hyde

Broadbottom

Ryder Brow

Reddish North

Hyde Central

Glossop

Manchester Oxford Road
short stay only

Levenshulme

Trafford Bar

Mauldeth Road

Heaton Chapel

Brinnington

Woodley

Burnage

Bredbury

East Didsbury

Romiley

Stockport

Gatley

Davenport

Rose Hill

Marple

Cheadle Hulme

Woodsmoor

Strines

Hazel Grove

Middlewood

Heald Green

Bramhall

Disley

New Mills Central

Handforth

Poynton

New Mills Newtown

Styal

Furness Vale

Wilmslow

Adlington

Whaley Bridge

Chinley

Crewe, Shrewsbury & South Wales

Crewe & London Euston

Macclesfield, Stoke-on-Trent & London Euston

Buxton

Sheffield

USEFUL INFORMATION

Getting around

Combined bus, train and tram journeys

DaySaver tickets let you make as many journeys as you wish at off-peak times using a combination of buses, trains and trams. The DaySaver ticket range lets you choose which combinations of travel you want. Buy a DaySaver at the bus driver, station ticket office (or conductor on the train if closed) or tram stop ticket machine before you make your first trip.

Full details are available from www.gmpte.com, GMPTE Travelshops or by phoning Traveline on 0871 200 22 33.

Finding out more from GMPTE

There are GMPTE Travelshops at all major bus stations in Greater Manchester. Travelshop staff can help you plan your journey for buses, trains and trams; and can provide free timetables, maps and other leaflets you may need. They will also give you independent advice about the best tickets available for your journey.

Information is displayed at most bus stops and tram stops, and at bus and train stations.

www.gmpte.com also has all the information you need, complete with a journey planner, maps of the area and timetables for individual services to download.

You can also phone Traveline on 0871 200 22 33 where you can get information and advice about all the services available. The lines are open between 7am and 8pm weekdays and from 8am on weekends and public holidays.

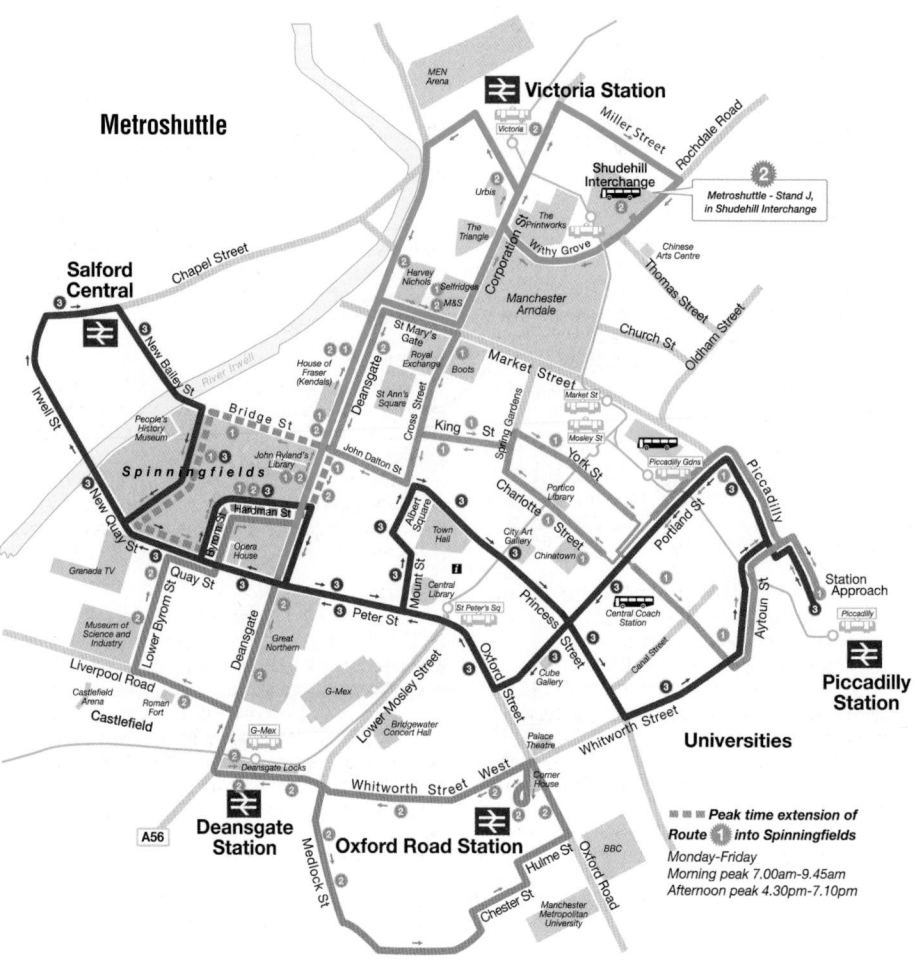

USEFUL INFORMATION

Even a seasonal traveller can find air travel with children stressful. Hopefully this information might help get your trip off to a relaxing start.

Manchester Airport

Manchester Airport is currently being upgraded at a cost of £80 million. Work should be completed by the summer of 2009. Landside facilities have been reduced, with investment being made airside, including an overhaul of security. The aim is to make your passage through the airport as fast and stress free as possible as it's this area that has been found to worry people most.

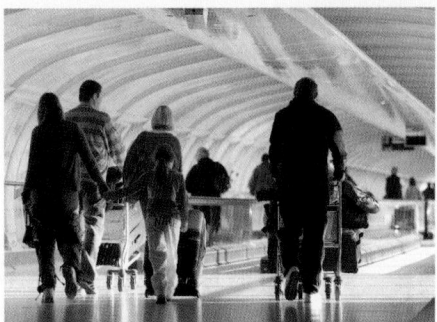

Getting there

To make things easier when you're travelling with children, allow yourself plenty of time for everything, from parking the car to walking to the gate. Manchester Airport is supported by excellent road and rail links and the train station is connected to Terminal 1 by a walkway. Buses and trains run 24/7.

If you're driving to the airport, pre-book a car park as it's considerably better value. Either call or book online.

The best value parking option, the Shuttle Park, is also the furthest away with a 15 minute bus transfer. Premier Park is a 5/10 minute transfer and the Long Stay car park is a 5 minute transfer. Alternatively you can pay extra and park in the Short Stay car park and walk into the terminal. For complete indulgence there is also Valet Parking. Based directly next to the Terminals it is just a few minutes walk to the check-in desks. If you can splash out it makes it a much less stressful start to your trip, especially if you're travelling with children.

In the Terminal

You can take your buggy all the way to the gate. It'll be useful to keep it with you in case toddlers need a nap, you're delayed or just to carry all the extra stuff that you end up not using! There are new pushchair friendly channels leading through to security making things a little easier.

If you are taking baby food or milk, it must be in a re-sealable container and you will have to taste it before going through security. These can be any size.

Any liquids or creams must be 100ml or less if you're carrying it in your hand luggage but Boots is located after security in all terminals so you could purchase items here to carry-on with you. In Terminal 1 I spotted four different brands of baby milk in cartons and a variety of baby jars. You can also stock up on medicines and sun cream.

Baby changing facilities in Terminal 1 have been upgraded to include a soft padded changing mat, a children's high chair, a bottle warmer and a breastfeeding area. In Terminals 2 and 3 baby changing is by the ladies toilet.

Upstairs on the mezzanine floor on Level 2 of Terminal 1 there is an enclosed children's play area, with a TV showing cartoons and a table with colouring pens. Bottle warmers for milk and food are available. Terminal 2 are currently undergoing a complete overhaul which should be completed by the summer.

If you want a bit of luxury, there are two lounges that allow children; the Bollin Lounge in Terminal 1 and the Styal Lounge in Terminal 2. They offer complimentary drinks, snacks, newspapers and magazines. It costs £17.95 per person and you have to pay full price for children of any age.

If you have some time and want to watch the planes, the Spectator's Terrace is located at Terminal 1 on Level 13 of the multi-storey car park.

Available throughout the airport and in most café areas are hot spots for laptops. This is also a good place to charge up any dvd players before a flight. As my family are confirmed TV addicts, this is an essential item in my hand luggage!

Eating

The Real Food Company, in Terminal 1, offers a child's meal such as half a jacket potato with filling or beans on toast plus a drink for £1.99. Lunchboxes are £2.99 with a choice of five items: a sandwich, jelly, fruit, crisps, chocolate bar and drink. Also here you will find Giraffe (review on page 56) where there are mezze plates for sharing and children's meals including an all day brunch or grill for £3.95 and delicious smoothies for £2.10.

Finally...

Families are usually invited to board the aircraft first, but if you've got a seat booked, I see little point in extending the time spent on board with a restless baby or toddler and as a general rule I try and get on last!

It's worth contacting your airline before you travel, to see what they provide on board for children, such as sky cots, baby food, toddler meals, and any children's entertainment. If you're travelling on your own with small children, also enquire to see what extra help they can offer.

Manchester Airport, Manchester M90 1QX
Tel: 08712 710 711
Car Park Mon-Sun 7am-10pm Tel: 0871 310 2200
Executive Lounge Tel: 0870 787 6877
www.executivelounges.com
www.manchesterairport.co.uk

USEFUL INFORMATION

Index

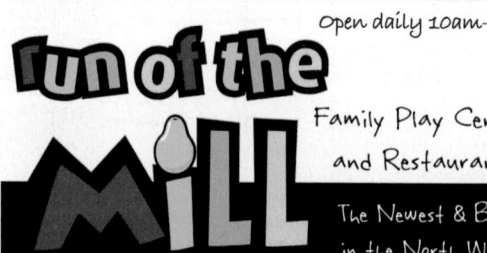
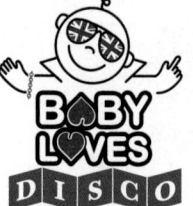

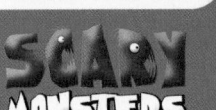
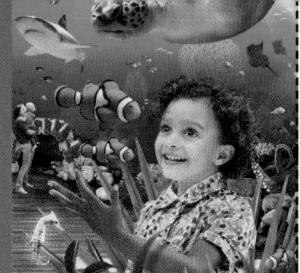
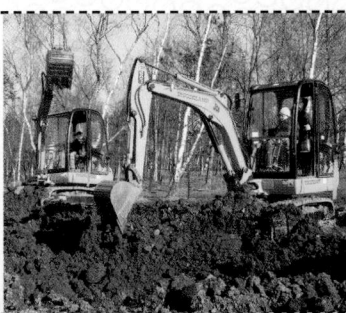
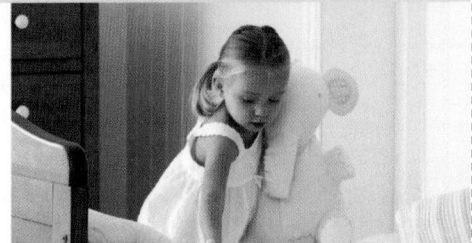

Index

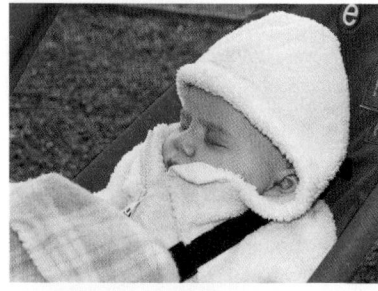

Babies in the City

Babies in the City would love to hear from you about the places you and your family enjoy visiting or where you like to eat.

Email us with photos of your favourite day out and the best ones will go on our website and possibly even in the 2010 edition!

Keep checking our website for regular updates.

info@babiesinthecity.co.uk
www.babiesinthecity.co.uk

By entering your details you will be kept up to date with the latest news and offers and also receive £5 off in store.

Title: _____ First name: _____ Surname: _____

House No.: _____ Address: _____

Postcode: _____

Baby's due date/ Birthday: _____ dd / mm / yy Email: _____